This HOUSE SMELLS LIKE FARTS

*a memoir of love,
loss, & getting on with life*

MEGAN JONES

Year of the Book
135 Glen Avenue
Glen Rock, PA 17327

ISBN: 978-1-64649-330-2 (paperback)
ISBN: 978-1-64649-342-5 (ebook)

Printed in the United States of America

Dedication

To my mom and dad

The day my husband died, my parents put their lives on hold. They were busy enjoying their retirement after many hardworking years. They were already active grandparents to four grandsons, yet they still found time to do things for my grandmother. This all came to a halt that Sunday morning.

When I realized the inevitable, that my husband wasn't coming home from the hospital, I looked at Mom and said, "What am I going to do?" And like so many times in my life, she simply said, "It will be okay." In the past, even when I had been sure that it really would not be okay... it always was. She was always right. So I trusted her now.

My parents have made me the best version of myself and I continuously learn from their generosity and love. I am so fortunate to be a recipient of their unconditional love, and I hope that in some way I can replicate what they have done for me.

Introduction

May 2023

When my oldest son was diagnosed with autism, I felt so many emotions. In a way, I think I went through all the stages of grief. When I finally reached acceptance, I also knew the reason I was chosen to be Oscar's mom. He makes me strive to be a better person. I try to intentionally be more patient with all people, regardless of their intellect or capability.

I know you are only given in life what you can handle. At the time of my husband's death, I felt like I already had enough on my plate. In a way I felt like I was in a choose-your-own-adventure book, and I had inadvertently chosen the hardest adventure. Unfortunately there was no going back to the beginning of the story to choose a different journey.

I know everything happens for a reason. I will never fully understand why my time with Wally was cut short. I have decided that I will live my life with purpose and positivity. I will celebrate when I can. I will give myself grace to make mistakes. Most importantly, I will remain obsessed with my sons and the unconditional love I feel for them.

1

November 2018

I was so excited to get an extra hour of sleep. It was November and the end of daylight savings time. No one warns you when you have kids that the days involving springing forward and falling back are a nightmare. And if you are lucky enough to have an infant that does not yet sleep through the night, during the end of daylight savings you are in for an extra treat, because babies get up whenever they want, and need to eat whenever they want. So instead of getting that famous *extra* hour of sleep in the autumn, parents of infants are blessed with a twenty-fifth hour in their day.

My days already consisted of making decisions from 7:00 A.M. until 9:00 P.M. ... decisions about what clothing everyone would wear, decisions at work, decisions for children, decisions about what to make for dinner, and finally, decisions for myself. Now that my sons were five and seven years old, at least I was finally able to appreciate the extra hour of decision-free sleep.

We had celebrated the boys' birthdays the night before with family and a few of our younger son Harvey's friends. I cleaned up a bit and went to bed shortly after my husband Wally, deciding we could take care of the rest in the morning.

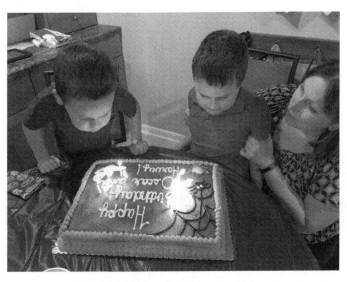

Oscar and Harvey's birthday party in 2013,
the day before Wally passed away.

I woke up at 5:30 when my husband grabbed my arm. He took a huge gasp of air. I remember asking him if he was okay. The last thing he said was, "I don't know."

Then he stopped breathing. He started turning blue. One of the most surreal things I have ever experienced is not feeling my husband's heartbeat when I took his pulse. I called 911 as fast as I could.

I woke up at 5:30 when my husband grabbed my arm.

The 911 operator asked if I could safely move Wally to the floor and put her on speaker so she could help me. I literally shoved and pulled my husband off the bed. I remember kicking him with both my legs to get him to the floor.

The operator told me to start chest compressions. After that didn't work, I started mouth-to-mouth resuscitation. I know it didn't take long for the paramedics to arrive, but it felt like forever. I remember thinking that when they got to our house, they would be able to do something I hadn't been able to—they would be able to turn things around.

I thought the paramedics would be able to turn things around.

I kept going with CPR until I was interrupted by a small voice behind me.

"Mommy?"

All of the commotion had woken our youngest son who is an early riser to begin with. I yelled at Harvey to go back to his room.

After what seemed like forever, the ambulance arrived. At the time, our family had a year-old dog named Johnny Cash—the dog in black. He loved people and got excited when anyone came to the door.

Unbeknownst to me, paramedics won't enter your house if your dog is not caged or restrained. I chased Johnny Cash into the basement and let the paramedics know it was safe to enter. As they took over compressions, I sat on our bed trying to wrap my mind around what was happening.

After a few minutes, I called my parents. One of the reasons we had moved into this house in York, Pennsylvania, was because it was in the same neighborhood where I grew up. My parents thankfully lived just down the street.

I brought Mom up to speed and she let me know she was on her way.

Everything during that time was such a blur. I know the paramedics were only at my house for a short period of time but it dragged like an eternity.

"Ma'am?" My racing thoughts were interrupted by one of the paramedics trying to get my attention. He motioned to the door and there stood my youngest son again, taking everything in.

I quickly moved him out of the room.

During this time my mom arrived. She was coming up the stairs from the living room just as I was trying to get my son out of the way of the paramedics. I tried to tell her as much as I knew.

I was prepared for the worst possible outcome... and I needed to share that worry.

I was prepared for the worst possible outcome... and I needed to share that worry.

"He died?" she asked. It was almost a whisper. I don't think she believed it, and she also didn't want my son to overhear.

Since no one really prepares for this conversation, my response was so very odd. "Well, not yet." I think I was hoping the paramedics would be able to wave some sort of magic wand like on a medical drama.

The paramedics came out of our bedroom and said they were taking Wally to the hospital. We moved out of the way, and I got myself ready to ride in the ambulance.

It's definitely not a good sign when the paramedics tell you to have someone else drive you to the hospital instead. It didn't sink in until much later that they do that so you don't have to watch what happens when they try to resuscitate someone.

> *It's not a good sign when the paramedics tell you to have someone else drive you to the hospital.*

My mom called my dad with the hope that he could drive me to the hospital. But when he got to my house and we updated him, it became obvious that I would need an alternative method of transportation.

My father can at times appear stoic, but when it comes to the happiness of his family he melts faster than an ice cube in the summer sun.

One of the paramedics had been my high school band instructor. He volunteered to drive me. After one more attempt to convince everyone I could drive myself, I gave in and accepted the ride.

2

April 2010

My husband and I met in high school. I was a freshman and he was a senior.

It was the first week of band camp, and I had no idea what to expect. I went into the band room to put on my snare drum for morning rehearsal.

Wally played the trumpet and was talking to another person from his section. Incidentally that person was dating my cousin so he said hello to me as I came into the room.

Wally made a comment about me being a girl drummer and how cool that was. We interacted a few more times during the next two weeks and then school started.

On the way home from our first away game, a random girl, who I only knew in passing, came up to my seat and asked if I wanted to move to the back of the bus to sit with Wally. As a freshman, this was a pretty big deal. The hierarchy of seating on a band bus is learned very quickly.

A week or so later, Wally asked if he could call me. This was well before the age of cell phones so a personal call meant taking the landline rotary phone and trying to create some type of privacy. Thankfully my parents were kind enough to let me use the phone in their room and I only had to navigate interference from a nosy younger sister.

A personal call meant using the landline rotary phone in my parents' room for privacy.

I was fifteen years old and not allowed to date. Too embarrassed to tell Wally, I didn't want him thinking that asking me out would be our next step.

We finished that year of school, Wally graduated, and we didn't talk again. I had no idea what his future plans were or if he was going to college. I appreciated our interactions for what they had been—a young crush that I would eventually get over.

Flash forward 15 years. Facebook enters the world and suddenly we can connect with people we haven't seen in over a decade. At some point, Wally and I became Facebook friends. I'm honestly not sure who friended who. But I remember the way I felt when I received a message from him. I was suddenly that flattered high school girl all over again.

We messaged each other back and forth a few times. I assumed he was just being friendly until he invited me to see a movie with him at the theater where he worked, about an hour away. I was skeptical and remember asking him if he was going to join me or if he would be working the whole time. Looking back now I realize what a silly question that must have seemed like.

But our plans fell through, and we decided to do something closer to where I lived. Wally picked me up on his motorcycle and we went for a short ride before stopping for dinner.

We had a great conversation. We laughed a lot, which became a theme in our marriage. Then we took another ride before he dropped me off at home. He even came inside and watched television with me and my roommate.

Wally didn't stay long though. He still had an hour drive home. I thought it had been a great date, let alone a great *first* date.

When he left, I walked him to the door, and before I could decide if I wanted to give him a hug, he stuck out his hand for a handshake. This completely caught me off guard. We had been inches apart on his motorcycle for at least half of our time together. The idea of a handshake left me dumbfounded.

I immediately second-guessed what my idea of a good date must be. I went to bed feeling like I had misread the entire situation.

When he left, he stuck out his hand for a handshake.

Then I woke up the next morning to a text message from Wally about how much fun he had, saying that he hadn't laughed like that in a long time, and that we definitely needed to hang out again.

It's at this point that I realized how different this date had truly been. Thank goodness for that handshake. It really did change my life.

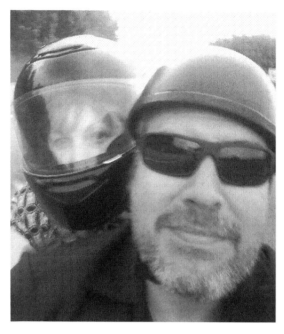

*This was not taken on our first date, but rather on a date night.
If it was nice weather, we always tried to take the bike.*

3

November 2018

When I arrived at the hospital, we went into the emergency department. I told the receptionist that my husband had been brought in by ambulance.

It wasn't long before I was taken into a small room with a family liaison. Then that woman brought in the hospital chaplain. It became obvious to me that the news was not going to be good.

After everything that happened at the house, it was what I had expected. But I was still holding out some type of hope that things were not so bleak. Or at least that I wouldn't have to make a life-or-death medical decision about what would happen next. I knew what Wally wanted, but selfishly if a doctor told me he was alive, I wanted to keep him that way no matter what.

I remembered having a conversation with Wally when I was in labor with our first son. There are so many things that can go wrong during delivery. When it was time to push, my nurses were intense cheerleaders. I was excited to meet my son but also scared of the delivery process.

I grabbed my husband by the arm. Words tumbled out nonstop. "If I need to have a C-section and I have surgery, and something happens, don't let me be a vegetable. But also don't let me die. Whatever happens, just don't let the baby die." It was quick but cemented the fact that Wally knew my wishes.

When the chaplain was brought in, it was obvious the news was not going to be good.

When the ER doctor joined me and the chaplain and the family liaison, he told me that despite everything they had attempted, they could not resuscitate my husband.

Part of me was grateful I wouldn't be forced to make the life-or-death decision.

There would be plenty of other painful decisions headed my way.

Before the doctor took me to see Wally, the chaplain told me, "When you see your husband, stay as long as you need to. There's no rush. Take your time. You can grieve there. You can break down. When you leave, you will be on autopilot. You won't let yourself fall apart."

I sat by Wally's bed and just cried and talked to him. The chaplain's words kept ringing in my head. She had said that when I left that room I would be on autopilot. I would go through the motions of life and make sure everything worked for my boys.

> *In that hospital room, time*
> *would stand still for me.*

I understood in that moment, more than anything, that in that hospital room time would stand still for me. I wouldn't have to worry about telling my sons their father had died, or worry about planning a funeral.

I knew eventually I would have to leave that safe space, but I wanted to stay there as long as I could before I had to deal with reality.

4

June 2010

Wally and I decided to get married in the Outer Banks where my family had vacationed several times. Other than knowing we wanted to get married, we knew nothing about what was involved in actually planning a wedding.

There was only so much we could do before arriving. Once we reached North Carolina, we got the marriage license before dinner and planned to head to the district magistrate the next morning.

We arrived at the Dare County District Magistrate's office bright and early on a Tuesday. Conveniently located next to the county detention center and across the street from the garbage truck parking lot, the location made sense for overseeing police and criminal activity... but for a marriage it seemed humorous to us. Then again, laughter was already a big part of our relationship.

"So we're getting married in jail?" Wally chuckled.

As we waited, we saw two policeman escort a teenager into the detention center. The boy was barefoot, shirtless, and looked like he had spent the night on the beach getting into trouble. A woman and younger girl also came in. At the time I assumed it was probably the mom and sister.

All of this of course put a delay on our "ceremony."

The Magistrate's office was conveniently located next to the county detention center.

Wally was quiet. Too quiet. I could see the delay was making him anxious. Or maybe it was being trapped in a small room with my parents, not to mention my sister, her husband and their child.

When it was finally our turn with the magistrate, he came out of his office and opened a door that led into a conference room. Our ceremony lasted all of ten minutes. We didn't even have our rings at the time.

On our way back to the house, we stopped at the Wright Brothers Museum at Kitty Hawk and at a jewelry store to purchase rings.

There was nothing traditional about our month-and-a-half engagement, our wedding day, or our reception back home in Pennsylvania. I wouldn't recommend it for everyone but it worked for us.

The tale of our wedding was a story I would overhear my husband tell again and again. He would always start with the punchline, "We got married in jail." After seeing a confused look on the listener's face, he would proceed to tell them about the beach bum who preempted our ceremony.

Wally joked, "We got married in jail."

Part of the reason our lives worked so well together was that we always saw the humor in day-to-day activities. I'm glad our wedding day was no exception.

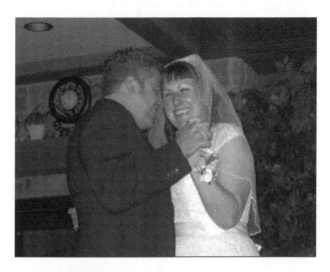

Our wedding reception, October 2010.
It took place four months after our actual wedding,
but was such a fun day.

5

November 2018

The morning Wally passed away, I entered a surreal time. I was aware this was the start of a new life for my family.

Dad picked me up from the hospital and we drove home in complete silence. He was just as upset as I was. Partially, I think it was because he was so fond of Wally, but also because it takes a toll on you to see your child in so much pain. I've had a lot of those same thoughts on behalf of my sons who are going through life without their father.

When I got home, Harvey came to me and I had to tell him what happened. Keep in mind this five-year-old had seen the paramedics come into our house and take his father away.

I started off with, "Harvey, I need to tell you something about Daddy."

Without missing a beat Harvey asked, "Did he die?" He has always been, and continues to be, so perceptive. He completely caught me off guard with his response. I was at a loss for words. "Did he die?" he asked again.

I couldn't bring myself to say anything so my mom had to jump in. "Yes, honey. He died."

"Did he die?" Harvey asked.

Harvey wanted to know how his dad died, and I explained as best I could to a young boy what happens when someone has a heart attack. I have always tried my best not to sugarcoat anything for him. I've found that being honest works best.

I said, "Well, sometimes people have something happen to their heart, and their heart stops beating. And it doesn't start again."

Over the next few months Harvey would tell others, sometimes random strangers, that his dad died. That his heart had stopped *beeping*. Yes beeping. Keep in mind he was five at the time. I think when he retold the facts to people it was his way of processing everything. The more he said it, the more it sunk in, and the more real it became.

Harvey still has days when he is especially upset about something, and will say he misses his dad or he wants his dad. I know those feelings will never go away. I wasn't fortunate enough to meet my father-in-law, but I remember having similar moments with Wally. He would simply state that he missed his dad and wished he was there to answer a question or show him how to do something.

I know I have more of these kinds of days ahead with Harvey where he will wish his dad was here to answer a question or just give him a hug and encouragement. I feel the same way and hope I can help guide him through those feelings.

I never told Oscar.

I never told Oscar. I don't know if it was because I didn't think he would understand. *Or...*

6

July 2011

When I was seven months pregnant with our first son, Oscar, Wally and I took our weekly trip to the grocery store. We almost always had the same routine. Wally would push the cart and I would man the shopping list and organize coupons.

I would give him things to find and he would add anything to the cart that he wanted that wasn't on the list. I definitely had the more exciting part of the task.

Occasionally he would lose interest or something would catch his eye if I took too long to find something. We were in an aisle that wasn't easy to navigate. Out of the corner of my eye, I saw Wally stop and head toward one of the displays.

Our grocery store, like most, has gadgets and toys hanging in the middle of other items to entice you to buy things you otherwise wouldn't know you needed. This display had mass quantities of super balls. Each bag had about 25 balls in it.

I watched Wally as he picked up the bag and examined it. He turned it around in his hands and I knew exactly what he was thinking. "If one of these balls bounces *this* high... how high would the *entire bag of balls* bounce?"

I watched Wally pick up the bag of balls...

I really appreciated how his brain worked. Before I could stop Wally, he raised his hands slightly and dropped the bag onto the floor. I think he was honestly expecting its contents to bounce twenty feet into the air. Instead the bag broke open and all the balls exploded down the aisle and into the common area.

We both immediately started laughing. If I remember correctly there was an "Oh shit!" from Wally and I rushed to the bathroom—because at this stage of my pregnancy there were never enough potty breaks. I was fully aware that releasing my bladder in the middle of the store would bring more attention to the super ball disaster.

When I finally got to the bathroom, still laughing, I had one thought. *Oh my God, I'm going to have two of them.* We knew at this point that we were having a boy and I could only imagine the antics my husband and future son would get into. I was convinced we would probably have more than our share of grocery store episodes like this.

> *I could only imagine the antics my husband and future son would get into.*

7

November 2018

After composing myself for what seemed like the tenth time that day, I realized I needed to get in touch with Wally's mom and his sisters.

His mother was local and would probably soon be headed to church. His older sister lived forty-five minutes away. I wanted her to be able to be with their mom after I told her. Wally's other sister lived in California, so I knew I'd be waking her up. Still, I didn't want her to hear the news secondhand.

I called Wally's oldest sister first, but she didn't answer. I left a message for her to call me back, and then I called the sister in California.

Everything had happened so early in the morning. I was already home from the hospital by 7:00 A.M. I don't know exactly what time I phoned, but she answered despite the time difference. I apologized for calling so early but once I told her why, she completely understood.

"I'm headed to your mom's. Could you check on her throughout the day?"

We were finishing up our conversation when his other sister called me back. I really didn't want to tell her over the phone about her brother. "I need you to go to your mom's house. I'll meet you there."

Her response was, "What's going on?" I know there was no way she could have expected what I was about to tell her. But after I did, she let me know that she was on her way to her mother's house. She was so shocked, as almost everyone was, when I shared the news.

When I arrived, his mom opened the door and said, "What did I do now?"

Wally's mom had been exhibiting signs of dementia.

The past few months had been tough for Wally and his sisters, as they tried to figure out their mom's next living situation. She had been exhibiting signs of dementia and it was becoming clear she shouldn't be living on her own.

"Nothing," I answered. "You didn't do anything wrong. I need you to sit down."

I explained what happened. "The paramedics and doctors did everything they could."

She opened the door and said, "What did I do now?"

No parent should ever have to be told this news.

A little while later his sister arrived and I told the whole story again. It wouldn't be the last time that day.

After a while, I felt like a broken record. I returned home to start making more of those calls, retelling the story. Each time it brought back all the painful memories from that morning.

8

February 2018

Wally and I didn't have a huge social media presence. We both had Facebook and Instagram accounts, but they were used more to connect with others or share a funny story. The two of us had a friendly competition about who could get the most likes or comments. With the addition of our newest family member—our puppy Johnny Cash—Wally thought he had figured out the secret algorithm.

"I really thought cute kid pictures were the secret ingredient in getting Facebook likes. But it's actually puppies. Wait a minute... what about puppies with cute kids?"

"I think you might be on to something," I replied. "If our kids get this many likes, and Johnny Cash gets this many, it just makes sense that the two combined would exponentially increase the number."

Walter Jones
Feb 15, 2016 · 👥

Ignore the messy living room and focus on the immense love this old dog has for his boy.

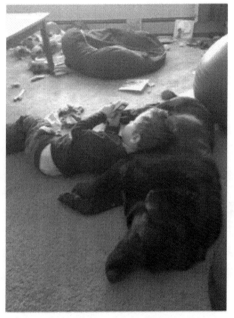

👍 You, Renaye Hoffman and 35 others   4 comments

Oscar and Shadow, our first dog.

And then I had the idea to also tag Wally whenever I made a post about the boys or the dog. That way his friends would also add to my likes and my win column. I didn't care if this was "playing dirty." It was all part of healthy competition.

Megan Jones is with **Walter Jones.**
Sep 18, 2018 · 👥

When kids dress themselves... they pick hand me downs that are over 30 years old.

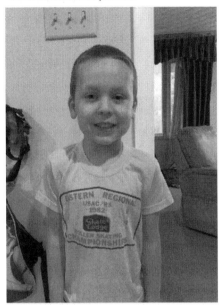

👍😮 Angie Persing and 40 others   5 comments

Harvey wearing his dad's old shirt.

9

November 2018

After I came home from Wally's mom's house, I knew my day would be consumed with countless phone calls. I gave his sisters the horrible task of informing that side of the family, and put my parents and sister in charge of reaching out to my family.

That left our friends up to me. Each time I made a phone call I relived the morning's events and what had happened. If I did manage to stop crying, it would start all over again.

There was no instruction manual for what you are supposed to do when your young spouse dies. I filled this day with countless cups of coffee and not much food. My parents stayed with me, and slowly the group at my house grew larger with more and more family members. Some brought food, asking what I needed, and others just stopped in to visit and keep me company.

My first phone call was to my manager. Keep in mind, I had only started this job seven months earlier. It was a brand new career for me. All they knew about me was what they had learned in the short time I worked there.

I don't remember a lot about that call. My boss and I cried through most of the conversation. I explained as much as I could about what happened. I asked her to let my coworkers know. I couldn't bear to tell the story more times than necessary.

Nothing affirmed my decision about having switched careers more clearly than when this same boss sent me a message the very next day asking, "What can I do for you today?" I knew this was not a work-related question, but just one human asking another what they could do to help.

She asked the same question the following day, and the day after that. Later that week, I met her and my office-mate for lunch and a much needed break from funeral planning. In the end I took a week off.

It was the first time since college graduation that I missed work for something unexpected. I was fortunate enough to be able to plan lawyer visits and other appointments around my work schedule. Remember when I said there are no instructions for this... there is so much involved after your spouse dies. It's overwhelming. Each event reminded me that I was now alone.

It was the first time since college graduation that I missed work for something unexpected.

My next call was to Wally's boss. I didn't have the phone number and I had never met him in person, so I needed to use Wally's cell phone to place the call. I know his boss was not expecting to hear my voice when he picked up the phone that Sunday morning.

He was shocked by what I told him. Wally had been there a little over a year, glad to finally not work nights or weekends and spend more time with family. From the number of coworkers who attended his funeral, I knew he was a valued employee. Of course I wasn't surprised. This was not a man that half-assed anything. Ever. Whether it was as a son, father, employee, or friend, you got 110 percent from him.

This made calling his friends so hard. Many had been friends since they were teenagers... decades. There is something absolutely unbearable about hearing grown men become emotional. I could never take it when it happened to my dad or my husband. Hearing his friends' sadness just confirmed what I already knew—Wally had been a wonderful friend who would have done anything for them and considered his close friends like brothers. It was amazing to witness that type of relationship.

After those big phone calls, I couldn't bear to tell the story one more time. I figured it would be safe to post a Facebook message to let everyone else know. It was so ironic that our relationship started via a Facebook message. I didn't want it to end that way, too.

It was so ironic that our relationship started via a Facebook message...

Wouldn't you know that this post would garner the most comments and notifications of my entire life. I think it was Wally's way of staying competitive in our little social media game.

Another joke between the two of us was my "black thumb" with plants. "Why would you even buy plants when you're just going to kill them?" he would ask. I still have two plants that I received during the week following his death. They have stayed alive for years despite my care. Instead of being a sad reminder, they are a tribute. I'm sure he has a hand in keeping them alive.

So many friends reached out after that Facebook post—friends from other states, friends I've known all of my life. I lost count of the text messages. I am thankful for all of them... like the friends who texted me because they were insomniacs and knew I wouldn't be able to sleep... the friends who brought food and entertained my sons... the friends who made me laugh and the friends who cried with me. They all have a special place in my heart.

In a way, Wally's death helped me become more connected. I started talking again to people I hadn't spoken to in years. I also think it made others appreciate their own relationships with their spouses a little bit more.

I've always been in the habit of saying, "I love you," to my family members when we finish a call or leave each other. After Wally passed away, I started doing this with my friends, too. If someone is important to you, you should tell them, because you never know when you may not be able to say it to them again.

10

December 2017

A year or two after Oscar was diagnosed with Autism, Wally and I were introduced to a financial planner who specialized in families with special needs children. His goal was to make sure families were set up for any circumstance in the future. He put us in contact with a lawyer who helped us write our wills.

Who knew that discussing numerous ways to kick the bucket would be so entertaining? The lawyer gave us scenarios and then we would decide in each situation who would raise the boys and who would be in charge of Oscar's care. The recommendation was that those people were not the same or married to one another.

I remember by the end of our session, my brain was all over the place. After being given another example of how I might enter the great beyond, I said, "Wait, who's dead now?"

Our lawyer shared our sense of humor and laughed with us as we went through each contingency plan. I had no way of knowing that in less than a year we would be reviewing Wally's will.

11

November 2018

It is not lost on me that funeral directors have one of the hardest and most thankless jobs. They see people on their very worst day and need to comfort them. But it is also their business and the way they make their living. It's how they put food on the table for their families. It takes a very special individual to make both of those things work. They make the family feel cared for while respecting the wishes of the deceased. They need to profit while not appearing to prosper from someone else's misfortune.

My funeral director was this special blend of human. Every step of the way he was compassionate and caring. He kept me notified and educated. There are so many things no one tells you about funeral planning and I never expected to be planning a funeral for my husband at the age of 42.

Wally and I had joked about our funerals to keep the idea of death light. We added detail after detail, each time trying to outdo the other's funeral spectacular.

I had a basic idea of what Wally would have actually preferred. I knew he wanted to be cremated and he was an avid motorcycle enthusiast. My funeral planner ordered a special gas tank urn.

Initially I didn't think Wally would have wanted the traditional church funeral but I changed my mind soon into my first meeting with the funeral planner. Mom came with me and his mom met us there. We picked out cards and poems, and honestly I'm not sure what else. The whole session was a blur.

At the end of our planning the funeral director asked the three of us if we wanted to see Wally one more time. My mom declined. I convinced his mom to go with me to say goodbye. He looked so peaceful. I think that was a moment that made everything real. I'm glad I did it. I needed to see him one last time to say goodbye. Seeing him like that didn't diminish any of my wonderful memories of him.

After the funeral home, I met with our church pastor to select hymns and scriptures. One of

Wally's joking wishes was to have a big marching band. We visualized a New Orleans street band playing "When the Saints Go Marching In" or a Southern gospel choir singing a hand clapping spiritual.

All jokes aside, I would love to have given him the marching band but I think we planned a service that would be a beautiful tribute to the caring father-son-husband that he was.

12

I called Mom to wish her a happy birthday. An hour later she called me back but it went to voicemail. When I was able to listen to her message later that morning I knew something wasn't right and I called immediately.

"Mom, what's wrong? What happened?"

Her voice was so shaky and I had never heard it like that before. "Uh, um, Pappy died this morning."

I had just been there the previous weekend for my sister's wedding and remembered seeing him and my grandmother dancing at the reception. They had been married 59 years.

That morning, my grandmother had been unable to wake him, so she called my mom and one of my uncles. They had both arrived at the same time as the ambulance.

Mom told me how the paramedics had tried to help. Ten years earlier, he had a massive heart attack and we had almost lost him. This time there wasn't anything that could be done.

"When we realized he was gone, your uncle Bob took a moment and said a prayer. I don't think I could have done that. And then Grandma remembered what day it was. She looked up at me and said, 'Oh Sharon, it's your birthday.' She didn't think about it until then."

A week later we all gathered in the same room where the bridesmaids and my sister had prepared for her wedding. This time for a funeral. The same preacher led us in prayer. The same group of people together for such different circumstances.

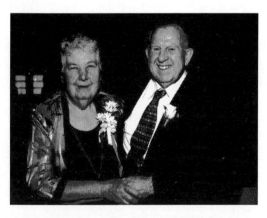

My grandparents, at my sister's wedding in 2005.
Grandpa passed away four days later.

13

November 2018

I was just so glad when there were no more phone calls to make. Then I received a call from one of my younger cousins. "Grandma and I are outside your house. Would you like some more visitors?" Hearing Wally's male friends cry had been bad enough. To see my grandmother get emotional would be my kryptonite... but I looked forward to her support.

The two of them came in, and of course the tears kept flowing. It had been thirteen years since her husband passed away. Over and over again, I wondered, *If I feel as bad as I do on this day, how much harder was it for Grandma to lose her husband after all that time together?*

You hear about couples losing a partner whom they've literally been with for half their life. Wally's death opened all those memories for her. Seeing her sadness made it all the more real for me.

This gave us a special connection that she didn't have with any of her other children or grandchildren. It's a connection I don't wish on any of my family members, but I also understand Grandma in a way I never could before. Her strength and ability to carry on alone has been something that keeps me moving forward.

14

October 2011

Oscar's due date was at the end of September, and it came and went. No one warns new moms the due date is only an approximation. Well, they probably do. But when you're so excited to have a baby, you don't really listen. Of course, by the end of the pregnancy journey you are really ready to not be pregnant anymore and that due date sticks in your head like glue.

On Oscar's due date I started to experience contractions. I had a scheduled appointment with my doctor and a test to make sure everything was still okay. At that point the doctor decided I should stop working.

I thought this was an excellent idea. Maybe the baby would come in a day or so, and if not, I would have time to clean and get ready. I could go for walks and spend time with Wally.

Even with all those possibilities, my anticipation got the best of me. I was so excited to meet my son.

After a week passed, the doctor set a date to induce labor. I was given instructions for what I needed to do, and I thought for sure that would be the day I would finally have this baby.

But here's another caveat... when you are induced, as long as you and the baby are still healthy, they really don't rush things. And if the hospital is full of moms in *actual* labor, you are put on the back burner.

Being told to call the hospital at 6:30 in the morning and thinking they would tell us, "Come on in!" was not realistic. They did however tell me to eat light throughout the day in case they were able to have me come in at some point.

After the previous nine months, this day was the hardest. There was simply nothing we could do. We were at the mercy of someone else.

We walked through our neighborhood numerous times that morning. As a nervous first-time mom, I kept calling the hospital to see if it was our turn yet. Finally Wally said, "Let's go get ice cream."

I'm not sure ice cream would be considered a light meal, but after only granola bars and yogurt, I was ready for some comfort food!

We went to an ice cream place and relaxed. I decided to call the hospital one more time, like a glutton for punishment. This time the nurse said she would check the status of rooms and call us back. It felt like progress. Finally some good news.

After the previous nine months, this day was the hardest.

We started to drive home and about ten minutes later the cell phone rang. The nurse asked us how long it would take for us to get to the hospital. In a blatant lie, my husband said, "Fifteen minutes."

Wally always wanted to have the opportunity to drive feverishly to the hospital in the hopes of being pulled over. Like in a movie he wanted to have to explain that his wife was in labor and we needed to get to the hospital *fast*. In his mind he would have a police escort and break all the speeding laws.

In this particular scenario though, his wife was not actually in labor. I'm pretty sure that "Yes officer, I know I was speeding but we have to get to the hospital before they give our spot away to someone else" wouldn't suffice.

When we did arrive at 3:30 that Friday afternoon, my midwife was already waiting. I was thankful for the ice cream sundae because at that point I was officially put on the ice chip diet. When my mom brought subs for dinner, I had to watch her and Wally eat them.

But the end result was wonderful. Oscar was born at 3:30 A.M. on Saturday.

That morning, after we were settled into our room, I had the biggest most amazing hospital breakfast!

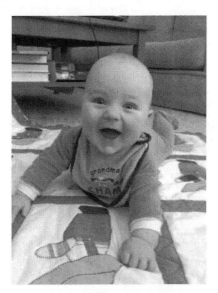

Oscar, 2012. A happy baby.

15

November 2018

The funeral was set for a Friday and I needed to return to work that following Monday. We all needed to get back to a sense of normal.

I sent the boys to school every single day except for the day of the funeral. I didn't want to disrupt their routines too much. Harvey was still in daycare, and Oscar was in first grade in an autism support class. Both schools were supportive and understanding.

I didn't take into consideration that on the day of the funeral I would still have mom duties. Not only did I need to get myself ready but also both boys. We arrived at the church just in time.

There were already people waiting to pay their respects. I met my husband's coworkers for the first time. I had heard so much about them, but it was nice to finally put faces with names, even under the circumstances. My current coworkers and past coworkers were also there. It was overwhelming how many people came through the line to tell me how sorry they were.

At the end of the visitation, the funeral director said, "That's it. You did great." The entire thing had been a blur.

"Do I have time to go to the bathroom?" I asked. I had been shaking hands and giving hugs for over an hour and needed a break before the service.

"Of course. Take as much time as you need. They're not going to start without you."

You can't start the funeral without the widow!

In a lot of ways a funeral director is like a wedding planner. This person sets the pace for the day and takes care of all the small details. My funeral director made sure I knew what was happening at any given time. He was meticulously organized.

This was probably one of the only funerals where the deceased's son looked at an iPad the entire time. I really just wanted Oscar to be as comfortable as possible.

It was a beautiful service. Lots of memories were shared. Looking back, I think Wally would have been happy with how it turned out.

At the end, the funeral director carried the urn with his ashes out of the church and the boys and I followed, the three of us linking arms.

Afterwards we had a luncheon that was made and served by the sweet and generous women from my church. This was the party Wally would have wanted. I visited with my friends, his friends, my parents' friends, and we all shared stories and memories.

The thing that would have made Wally most proud was that both of his sons were passing gas throughout the entire luncheon. Farts are funny in almost every situation, and oddly enough, a funeral is no exception.

16

Spring 2012

My husband's one love was motorcycles... or more specifically, anything with wheels and a motor. Okay, maybe it was a close second to his love for his family. But he loved motorcycles so much that I'm not sure there would have been a first date if I hadn't been comfortable riding with him. If that was his criteria for who he dated, so be it. It all ended up working out.

From our initial conversations I could tell that he had an enthusiasm for riding. It was a stress reliever and an outlet for him to clear his head. I was envious that he had something he felt that passionately about.

We never had less than two motorcycles in our garage at any given time. I truly believe he wanted a motorcycle for each day of the week.

Knowing about this passion, one would think that I would be super careful around any of his bikes, especially when in my car. And I was super careful. But not careful enough.

One day, I planned to run errands with Oscar, but when I backed out of the garage, my passenger side mirror clipped the mirror of Wally's motorcycle. It was just enough to set the bike off balance. In slow motion, I watched it fall to one side and hit the grass.

I moved with the speed of a ninja to see what damage I had done. Instinctively I got one shoulder under the bike and set it upright.

Then I realized I needed to call Wally and confess what had happened.

I started talking super fast to try to get everything out. "I knocked your bike over and I'm sorry. I picked it up—seems okay, no dents, just some grass on the foot pedals."

Wally paused for a long time and then said, "Wait, you picked up the motorcycle? Megan, that bike weighs six hundred pounds. How did you pick it up?"

"Wait, you picked up the motorcycle?"

Later he revealed to me the conversation he had with one of his coworkers. "I'm not sure if I'm more angry or afraid of her. It's not every day that your wife deadlifts a motorcycle."

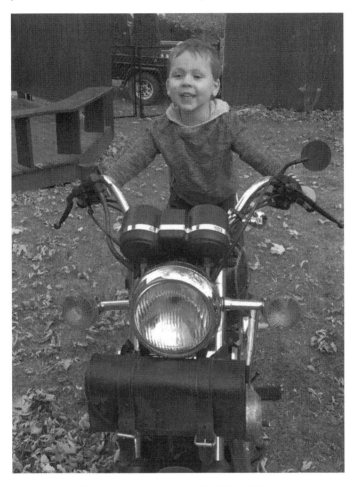

Harvey posing on one of Wally's bikes.

17

December 2018

After Wally's death in early November no one expected the holiday season to be joyful. I tried to stay upbeat for Harvey and Oscar. I wanted their Christmas to be as unaffected as possible, similar to past holidays.

When I decorated, I hung all four of our Christmas stockings. My mom had decided not to hang any of her own stockings, realizing that every time I saw them it would be a reminder.

Christmas Eve is by far my favorite church service. I love the pageantry and hymns, and the candlelight singing of "Silent Night." I remember being at that service over the years, watching people wipe tears from their eyes during that final hymn. Everyone remembers their lost loved ones in a different way. I never imagined that I would be one of those people holding back tears for my husband.

Normally after the service, Mom would go to my grandmother's house to help her prepare the turkey for Christmas Day. But that year, Grandma was adamant that Mom needed to come to my house. So she helped me put the boys to bed and offered to stay longer to help put gifts out, just like she told me she could spend the night the day that Wally died.

I let her go, for the same reason I had let her go on that first day. It was the same reason that I didn't have the nurses take Harvey to the nursery after he was born so I could get some sleep. I have always had a "rip the band-aid off" mentality. I would much rather just jump into whatever is inevitable.

The day that Wally died, I ripped off the largest band-aid ever. No matter how painful a day might be, I knew I would get through it, because that is what my husband would have wanted for his family. That is the faith that he had in my strength.

18

October 2013

I woke up on a Sunday and felt just a little off. I was uncomfortable but I had never experienced regular labor pains, so I continued on with my day. I went to work that night as planned. I had contractions most of the night but nothing I couldn't handle. I sent Wally text messages with updates. I don't think he believed me until I got home and found out for himself that my contractions were less than five minutes apart.

Anyone who has ever worked in a restaurant knows that you carry whatever food you made or served that night home with you as your new scent. When I got home from the restaurant, all I wanted was to take a shower so the baby wouldn't smell like fajitas. Based on how close my contractions were, the shower would have to wait.

We grabbed bags and Oscar and headed to the hospital. We were pulling out of our development when Wally became very quiet.

"Is something wrong?" I asked him.

I was getting ready to birth a human any moment. Part of me was annoyed that Wally seemed upset about something. I was close to losing my cool, when he finally answered, "I'm just focusing on my breathing."

I realized he had been joking the entire time.

Even when I was in excruciating pain, he could make me laugh. That was just what I needed. We arrived at the hospital at 1:00 A.M. and Harvey was born around 6:00 that morning.

Harvey has recently started asking me to tell him about the day he was born. He also wants to hear stories about when he was a baby. He asks over and over, "How did you feel?" It's such a hard question to answer, so difficult to put into words. It may sound cliché, but the happiest moments in my life were welcoming my sons into the world.

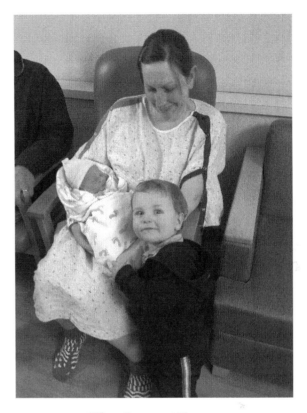

When Oscar met Harvey.
(This was the photo Wally used
as a screen saver on his phone.)

19

Summer 2019

That first year after my husband passed away, I wasn't sure how to handle the celebrations. I didn't want them to be sad memories for myself or for the boys. Wally and I had always made it a point to celebrate birthdays and our anniversary and I wanted to still carry on the tradition.

The first milestone that came up was the anniversary of our first date. It was April Fool's Day. On our actual date we didn't think anything about it being April 1st. Now I realize how fitting it was, since we had lots of laughter and never took ourselves too seriously.

My husband was also a generous person and would help anyone if he could. In that spirit, I decided to treat my staff to pizza for lunch. Not a grand gesture, but still something that people enjoyed. It gave me some comfort going through the day.

On Wally's birthday I donated blood to our local blood bank. He had been a frequent donor, and I felt like it was my job to take over for him. I looked at it almost as a tribute to all the times he had helped others. A month later, I received a letter saying that the blood bank had used my donation and had saved three separate patients, one of them an infant.

We had cake and ice cream on his birthday and I let Harvey invite one of his friends over. I'm sure it sounded strange to hear him say, "Do you want to come to my dad's birthday party?" to anyone who knew the situation. But Harvey didn't think anything of it. He still thought everyone had a party for their birthday. By that rationale, it would stand to reason that we would have a party for his deceased dad.

Our wedding anniversary was probably the hardest day of all for me. I tried to remember each of the happy memories from that first trip to the Outer Banks.

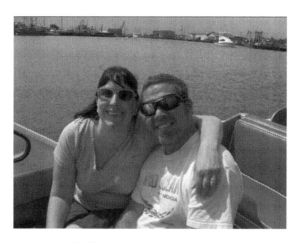

One of the first photos after we were married.
Outer Banks, 2010.

On the one-year anniversary of Wally's death, I took a personal day from work. I'm not sure I will ever be able to work on that day. Instead, I will celebrate all the amazing things about his life, and the wonderful legacy that he has in his two sons.

20

August 2013

When Oscar was eighteen months old, we took our first family vacation to the Outer Banks with my parents, my sister's family, and her in-laws. I noticed that my nephew, seven months younger than Oscar, was already saying words and interacting differently with people and toys. Oscar was always happy and easygoing, so I think Wally and I had just turned a blind eye to the fact that he wasn't doing things other kids his age could already do.

When we came home from vacation, I contacted our local early intervention department. They scheduled an appointment to evaluate Oscar in our home and also to have a conversation with us about our concerns.

I watched the evaluators and noticed their glances with each other. Oscar qualified for occupational therapy and special services. At the time I didn't understand what "special services" meant. Further into the process, I realized the instructors that had been assigned to him were well versed in therapies for children with autism. They had been chosen because the evaluators thought Oscar would likely be diagnosed with autism in the future.

Oscar's occupational therapist and special instructor came separately to our house once a week for 30 minutes. They knew each other and had worked together before. Occasionally they would come at the same time to work with our son.

When I was seven months pregnant with Harvey, the therapists asked if we would be taking a break from services once the baby was born. We hadn't realized that was even an option and wanted to do whatever would be best for Oscar.

When Harvey was born, we did take a week off, but the next week we were back on. Of course, the therapists were more than happy to hold a cuddly newborn so I could also participate in Oscar's therapy.

For the next year that's how we operated. As Harvey became older he was incorporated into Oscar's skills therapy and playtime. Even though we were not concerned about our younger son's development, the occupational therapist did an unofficial evaluation for Harvey just to put our minds at ease. In a lot of ways, it was like having a first child all over again. Harvey did things at ages that Oscar had not, and he mimicked his older brother's physical skills and quickly used those to learn how to walk, run, and scale many a chair or sofa.

Oscar officially graduated out of early intervention when he turned three years old. At that point he went to preschool through an intermediate unit program. His experience there was exceptional. I couldn't have asked for more.

I met with his occupational therapist and special instructor on his final day of therapy. They had become a part of our family. They had seen us every week, and watched both my sons grow. This was the first time I realized my journey with Oscar would lead me to meet great people who had the sole intention of helping others. I'm so thankful for early intervention and their support during this time.

21

September 2019

Getting three people ready every morning can be really hectic. Especially when those three people also have three different destinations. Oscar gets picked up by a van in our driveway and Harvey gets on the bus at his daycare. To save time, I back my car out of the garage into the driveway with everyone inside, ready to go.

On a perfect day the van picks up Oscar and I take Harvey to daycare and wait with him until his bus arrives. Sometimes the van is late, though, and we don't have as much time to get to Harvey's bus stop. Other times we are running late and I barely have the car in the driveway before Oscar's van pulls in.

On this particular day, everything was running right on schedule. I wanted to pat myself on the back. *I got this. We're gonna be okay.*

And then, the morning came to a screeching halt.

"I have to go the bathroom" came Harvey's small, nervous voice from the backseat.

"Is it just a pee?" I asked.

I got the response I was hoping for. "Yes. I think so."

It was a nice autumn day and while I am not an advocate for public urination, desperate times call for desperate measures. "Okay, just go behind the car. No one will see you."

Harvey was hidden by my car when he said, "I was wrong. It's a poop."

If there was ever a take-the-wind-out-of-your-sail moment, this was it. The morning had been moving right on track. Breakfasts fed, three people clothed and ready to walk out the door.

"Is it just a pee?" I asked.

Now, I need to figure out how to get my kindergartener into a bathroom while still watching for Oscar's van.

I reopened our garage door and told Harvey to run inside and use the downstairs bathroom. Not much time passed before he returned to the door that goes into the garage. His pants were by his ankles. Tearfully he said, "I couldn't open the door to the bathroom."

Nearly every door in my house is protected with a child lock. Harvey had become very good at using his tiny fingers to open said child locks. But this one, during his panic, was giving him trouble.

I assured him that everything would be okay and quickly followed him inside, knowing that at any moment Oscar's van might pull into the driveway.

"I was wrong. It's a poop," *he answered.*

We got to the bathroom and I heard his tiny voice behind me, pants still around his feet. "I didn't make it in time." In front of the bathroom was a perfect pile of poop. "I'm sorry, Mommy. I tried to make it. I just couldn't open the door in time."

I felt so bad for him, and then I realized he hadn't gotten any of his "accident" on his clothing, so we did a quick clean-up. The only trace of the crime scene was a small smudge on the back of his shoes which was easy to clean.

We headed back out through the garage to the car and made it just in time. Oscar's van arrived a few moments later.

I knew Harvey was embarrassed about his accident because it had been quite some time since anything like that had happened. But I also couldn't help but be impressed that he had managed to just squat on the floor and make no mess on himself.

The situation could have been so much worse. No one missed the bus that day. Everyone made it to where they needed to be, and I'm certain that when Harvey is older, we will both laugh at this story.

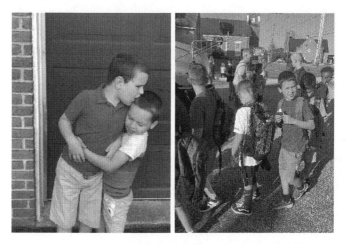

First day of school pictures.

22

February 2014

Wally and I drove to Baltimore with Oscar the night before Oscar's appointment at the medical center because there was snow in the forecast.

We'd had a previous appointment rescheduled because of a snowstorm. On that morning we had driven for over two hours and never made it out of our county. So we learned our lesson and booked a hotel this time.

The three of us arrived in Baltimore, checked into our room, had dinner, then settled in for the night. Even though it was already snowing, we were only ten minutes from the doctor's office. Falling asleep I remember thinking we had done everything right by staying overnight so close to the medical facility.

And we were early. So very early for that appointment.

Now that Oscar is older, I realize there is such a thing as arriving *too early*. His patience wears out and if what we are doing is not on his agenda, there is only a limited amount of time to accomplish the task at hand.

On this day, we waited over forty-five minutes for the developmental pediatrician to see us. By the time we actually saw the doctor, Oscar was on the verge of a full-blown meltdown.

There is such a thing as arriving too early.

The appointment was at the referral of his family pediatrician after we raised some developmental concerns at his well-child checkup. Oscar still had no consistent language, had stopped responding to his name, and no longer played with toys he once found interesting. When I saw other children that age and noticed how they played and interacted, I knew something was different.

We eventually ended up in an exam room after filling out a questionnaire about all things Oscar... his lack of development, his lack of socialization. The doctor came in and we went over the questionnaire and all the other reports from Oscar's other doctors. She asked more questions and observed him.

She spent roughly thirty minutes with us and after that time said she felt comfortable making a diagnosis of Autism Spectrum Disorder and Global Development Delay.

She gave us pamphlets, recommended tests we should do, and sent us on our way. I've never felt so unprepared. In my gut, I had known all along that this would be the diagnosis and outcome of the visit. Although Oscar was my first baby, I could tell he was different. Not a bad different... just different. He was so mellow. Almost too content. The only time he cried was when he was hungry. Those signs had been staring me in the face. Still, I was having trouble wrapping my head around what this meant for our lives.

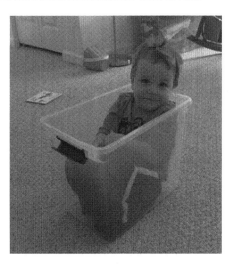

*We learned early on that Oscar
liked to be in tight, enclosed spaces.*

We got into the car for our drive home. My husband and I sat in absolute silence for what seemed like hours. After a few minutes Wally said, "At least now we know."

My response was through tears. "We are going to have the best damn kid with autism ever."

I still stand by these words. Yes, I have challenges with my son. I'm sure he feels he has challenges with me. But Oscar is such a blessing in my life. He teaches everyone he meets something different. He may drive you crazy and frustrate you, but his charisma and personality will forever wrap you around his finger.

23

October 2019

I never imagined that I would be attending Harvey's kindergarten orientation as a single parent. I had been to back to school nights for Oscar but this was something altogether different. Oscar's classes had been small and not the traditional learning environment or curriculum.

Harvey's back to school night was planned for both parents and their student. He and I went to visit his new classroom and meet his teacher. We learned about all the things he would do in his first year of school.

I was honestly overwhelmed. I hadn't had to worry about any of these things with Oscar. It felt like my first time, even though Oscar had already been in school for five years. I was getting anxious and nervous, and sitting at a small table on a tiny chair was not helping.

Then I met Harvey's teacher. This woman was exactly how you would imagine a kindergarten teacher should look. She seemed focused on building a foundation of learning for the children in her class. I knew immediately she was the right fit for Harvey. I made sure to be one of the last parents to leave.

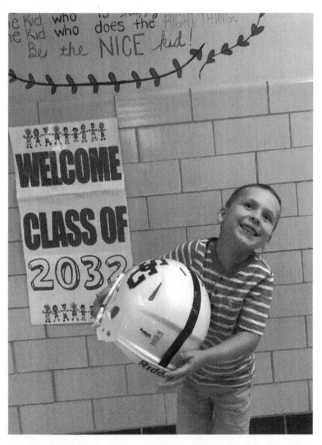

Harvey's kindergarten orientation picture - Class of 2032!!

While Harvey was entertained and playing, it gave me some time to talk to his teacher on my own. I explained our family situation to her and she was very understanding. I knew she would be patient with Harvey and would give him a great first year. She told me I could email her or call if I thought he was having a particularly rough day, or I if I knew there was something coming up that would make him think about his dad. She was incredibly compassionate, and I know she was pulling for Harvey and our family.

24

April 2015

When we first got married, Wally and I both had our own houses. His was close to where he worked but smaller than mine. We decided he would move in to my townhouse and commute to work, about a 45-minute drive while we rented his house to one of his friends. We lived there for almost three years together. In fact, both Oscar and Harvey came home from the hospital to that townhouse.

Wally and I knew that we eventually wanted a single-family home with room to grow. The housing development where I had been raised was built by my grandfather back in the late '70s. Two of my uncles lived there, nearby to my parents, and when a neighbor wanted to sell, I got a phone call.

The woman had long since moved out, and her two adult sons were now looking to move in different directions. The house was the raised rancher style that had been so popular in the '70s and '80s.

Wally and I were excited at the opportunity. I had such a great childhood in that peaceful neighborhood and wanted my boys to have similar experiences.

We made arrangements to see the house. Yes, it needed some work and it was a little outdated. It was also obvious that the two sons had not been the best housekeepers. But we could see through all that and knew we wanted to move forward.

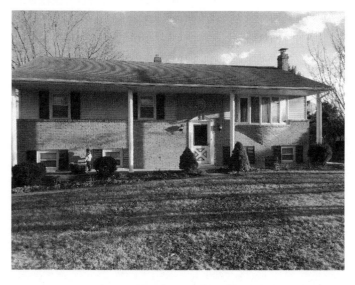

An outside picture of our house.

We felt slightly out of our minds to consider owning three homes, but decided to rent both our previous houses until the real estate market picked up again.

I have never experienced a closing on a house that has gone smoothly. This one followed suit. We were scheduled for a 1:00 P.M. meeting with the seller and all the important parties. But our new mortgage company had not given us the final amount.

We had assumed we could write a check at the meeting. Incorrect! This needed to be a cashier's check, but that bank was located forty-five minutes away. It was a race against the clock!

When we arrived at the bank in downtown Harrisburg, there were no parking spots. Wally circled city blocks while I raced inside. I had to stop myself from running out of the bank as well, realizing how suspicious that would look.

When we finally made it to our destination, the closing itself was smooth. Afterward, we treated ourselves to a late lunch and focused on making our new purchase our forever home.

Eventually I was able to sell the two houses that we were not living in. After a string of horrible renters in my house I was able to sell it roughly a year and a half after Wally passed away. His house was much easier. It went on the market fairly quickly. The man who purchased it was a single dad and his little girl loved the house. It made me so happy to be able to give them a fresh start as they were currently living with his parents.

We moved into our forever home right around Easter time. Harvey will still bring up the other house sometimes, which is odd because he wasn't even two when we moved. Occasionally he will ask me when we are leaving this house and I always tell him, "Never. We're staying here forever."

My parents actually live on the same street and it is a blessing to have them within walking distance. Without their help, our lives would look a lot different.

25

March 2018

When Wally and I were married, he had a dog and I had two cats. All three were in their later years and passed away early into our marriage. Once we were set up in our forever house and the boys were out of the toddler stage, we decided it was time to get another family pet. We knew we wanted to get a dog, and after talking to someone at work we found someone who was selling boxer Labradors. We 'adopted' Johnny Cash when he was eight weeks old.

He loved the boys. He had energy to run around with Harvey but was also content to lounge and be lounged on with Oscar. Wally took it upon himself to find a veterinarian for him and set up his initial appointment. He came home excited to tell me the story about how the vet technician called Johnny Cash's name and everyone in the waiting room remarked on his name and what a good looking dog he was.

After this vet visit, Wally decided that he would be the one to schedule and take Johnny Cash to all of his subsequent visits. He was oddly excited about this and compared it to something else.

"It will be just like when you take the boys to their well-child visits. I can schedule the appointments and make them around my work schedule."

I could tell how much he was looking forward to setting up everything and being in charge of Johnny Cash's health so I couldn't burst his bubble. I think he realized that A LOT more went into doctors' visits for two human children than a dog, even if it was an energetic puppy. And it was more than just generic doctors' visits. Oscar saw a speech and occupational therapist both once a week. He had additional services provided through medical assistance that needed to be set up periodically. There was a lot more coordination involved with setting up those appointments. I hated to state the obvious and take away the pride Wally had in his new task. I think this was also his way of taking something off my plate and not adding to it with another family member to take care of.

After Wally passed away, it was too much for our family to also have a pet. I felt like he was neglected and just didn't have the life he deserved. I reached out to a group that found homes for animals in similar situations. They found a wonderful family and Johnny Cash became their second dog. We joked that we had an open adoption because I became Facebook friends with the family and could watch Johnny Cash grow up. We spoke a year later after the family's older dog passed away. They said having Johnny Cash around helped them cope with their loss and brought them so much joy. I am so thankful that he found a home with them and I know Wally would approve.

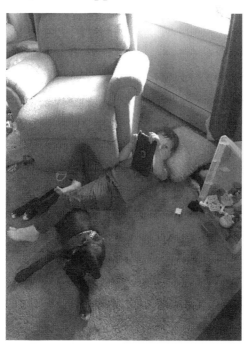

26

Summer 2021

Two years later I still forget that Wally's not here. More frequently the first year, something funny would happen and he would be the first person I wanted to share it with. Or I would just need to vent about work.

When I got promoted, I felt the loss immensely. I knew my parents and friends would be proud, but Wally would have been the most excited. He consistently supported me and would never let me doubt myself. "You're my rock," he would say, but the support was always mutual.

Recently I saw a brand of hard cider at the grocery store that I had only seen in the Outer Banks of North Carolina during our last vacation together. It was a local distributor there and we had enjoyed a variety pack. Seeing it reminded me of the beach and that trip, and took me back to memories of all our vacations. We had so many special times in North Carolina. After all, our marriage started there.

When I saw that label in the store, I had to stop myself from grabbing my phone and sending Wally a quick text. "Guess what I found?"

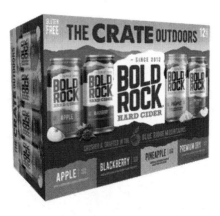

Our favorite cider in the Outer Banks.

I am so thankful that he was my person that I could text anytime, or call with a silly story. Wally always appreciated my humor. Our relationship had started out digitally as we used text messaging to catch up. After all, it had been eighteen years since we had last seen each other. I still feel a loss that I don't have that person.

Instead, I found I had people I could text for all different areas of my life. The friend I could text about work, the friends I could share a meme or pun, the moms (including my own mom) that I could vent to about parenting. In an odd way, not having a husband strengthened my relationship with many of my other friends and family.

No one will replace the unique relationship my husband and I had. But I'm not sure I ever realized what amazing people I had in my life until I needed to rely on them for their thoughts and correspondence.

27

Summer 2017

Whenever Wally and I received a tax refund, we made a plan for what to do with the money. A portion would go to our savings. Some would go into the boys' savings accounts, and finally we would each give ourselves an amount to purchase something fun or a splurge—something we wanted but wouldn't necessarily have purchased.

One year, Wally had decided he wanted to buy a fire pit. He had visions of building a fire after the boys were in bed and just spending time together, just the two of us.

While we did have some time alone, the most fun was when the boys would stay up late and we would roast marshmallows and make s'mores or pop popcorn over the fire.

We sometimes let Harvey help build the fire with smaller twigs and sticks. Oscar was never very interested, but would alternately sit with us for a while and then go back inside, eventually resurfacing for a snack.

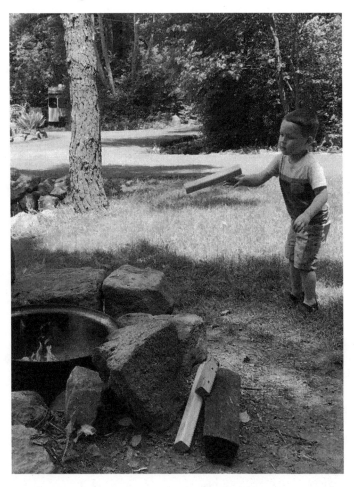

Harvey helping Dad with the fire pit.

One of our first family vacations was to a campsite that had custom-built cabins made out of nontraditional lodging. There were also places to set up tents or campers in addition to basic cottages for rent.

As far as the custom cabins... there was a teepee, a yurt, a double-decker bus, and a train caboose. At the time, Harvey was into all kinds of trains so the caboose was our obvious choice. It had two main rooms, a small master bedroom and another room that was the living area/kitchen/bunk beds.

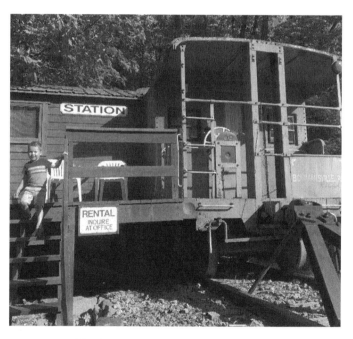

An outside picture of our caboose camping experience.

Each night we made our dinner over the fire or on the grill. Harvey wanted to help in any way he could and was excited to sleep in the bunk beds. He quickly climbed up to the top. He has always been a climber and has no concept that climbing could lead to falling. Some of his stunts literally took my breath away.

This was also my husband's birthday weekend so it was an extra special vacation. The campground was close to a nearby town, so on Wally's actual birthday, we went out for dinner and ice cream.

A different day, we took the boys on a paddle boat ride that neither one of them enjoyed. While I was doing my best to keep them both inside the boat, I neglected my paddling duties.

The campground also had a pool with slides and some water spraying features. The boys were a fan of this and we could all enjoy ourselves, unlike on the paddle boats.

We had such a fun time and talked about going camping again and eventually getting a camper. There was something so relaxing about the whole weekend that made us look forward to doing it again.

As it turns out, this would be the first and last time we went camping. We just never got around to planning another trip. In a way, I'm glad that I didn't have another trip to compare to the first one. We made memories that summer that I will always carry with me.

28

February 2020

On the first snow day of the year, I worked from home. My mom walked over to our house to help with online school for the kids. She knew there might be a future day when she would have to do this by herself, and she wanted to be prepared.

Three years had passed since the last big snowstorm. I hadn't touched a snow blower even though I was given an introductory lesson. I was also fortunate enough to have relatives living on my street who would dig me out if needed. Plus I had complete confidence in my driving ability with my four-wheel drive SUV.

The winter had been mild until the end of January. But in February we had several storms that caused school and work delays. This most recent storm started at night. By morning, schools were canceled with the intent that students would participate in online classes.

I had every intention of braving the weather and going to work, but as appointment cancelations continued to stream in, I realized I could be more productive working from home.

My workday started at 6:30 with calls, emails, and text messages. I had everything situated and a plan in place, ready to start the school day with the boys. My mom would help Harvey in the living room while I worked with Oscar in the kitchen. Sometimes we would work together to help them both.

Oscar signed on to his Zoom call scheduled for 8:00 A.M.[1] Because Oscar is nonverbal, he was not interrupting the teacher, but other students were. The session was very informal and even included breakout sessions where the teacher read a story to each of the students individually.

Oscar was clearly not in school mode. I think he was legitimately confused as to why his teacher was on his iPad. I spent most of the call chasing him around our kitchen, trying to get him to look at the camera. He did have a few giggles, and overall it wasn't a horrible experience.

We worked on the rest of his assignments together, and I submitted his work online to his

---

[1] If you ever have the opportunity to watch a Zoom class for autism support, I highly recommend it!

teacher. Later that evening she sent an email thanking me and my mom. She understood we had challenges, but apparently Oscar was the only student who had submitted any of his work that day, and she wanted us to know how much she appreciated that.

A first-grade Zoom class is equally entertaining. Harvey watched a video online for his music class before the first regular session. His teacher played the morning announcements. I was surprised that Harvey already knew how to use the mute button. I still have colleagues who struggle with this function.

Mom and I tried to make it as normal of a school day as possible. We all stood for the "Star-Spangled Banner" and I did my best to hit that high note with flair. It's like I had been picked to deliver the national anthem at the Super Bowl. Harvey's session consisted of a scavenger hunt with some instructions for the rest of the day.

Their classes continued while I attended my own meetings, keeping up with changing situations and schedules at work. At one point I looked up at Mom. "It's only 9:30."

By the afternoon, we had a much better flow going. Mom walked home for lunch and was gone for about an hour. The afternoon sessions resumed. She was a former elementary librarian and technology teacher, so I joked that I brought her out of retirement.

Like so many other days in my life, I'm not sure how I would have made it without her. She is patient and kind and does everything well, truly an inspiration and the biggest supporter and cheerleader in my life.

29

Winter 2017

We had our first big snowstorm in our new house the winter before Wally passed away. In previous years, we had no trouble making it out of the driveway. This snowstorm was different.

The forecast was for feet, not inches, over several days. On the first day, my restaurant and Wally's work both closed due to inclement weather. We were able to enjoy an actual snow day as a family.

Once I married Wally, I never had to worry about snow plowing or shoveling. He always cleared off my car if I parked outside. But to keep up with this storm, snow removal needed to be addressed multiple times.

When he finished plowing our driveway, he moved on to our neighbors. Then he went down the street and dug out my parents and another woman in the neighborhood. He was always willing to help anyone in need. Watching him that day made me proud to be his wife.

After all the snow cleanup, we took Harvey outside. He had never played in snow that deep. Oscar had a bit of a cough and was taking a nap, so it was a perfect opportunity for the rest of us to get outside.

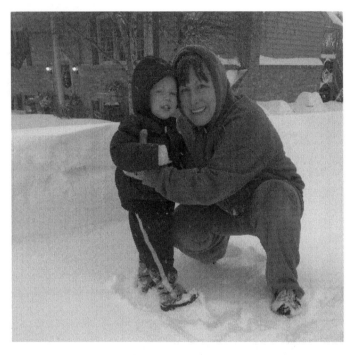

Megan and Harvey enjoying the snow.

The streets were still unplowed in our development so in some places we couldn't tell where our yard ended and the street began. We have pictures of Harvey standing in the middle of an intersection and you wouldn't be able to tell that it's one of the most traveled areas in our development.

It was just a relaxing day and so much fun to all be home together. Knowing that the next day's commute back to work would bring a huge headache made it that much sweeter.

30

September 2022

My son Oscar is one of the most perceptive people I have ever met. He is acutely aware of his surroundings at all times. The intriguing part is that he rarely seems to pay attention to anything going on. He may be watching television or a video on his phone, but he is always taking everything in, paying attention to slight differences and using those changes to his advantage. He will notice someone entering or leaving a room no matter how quiet or innocuous the person tries to be.

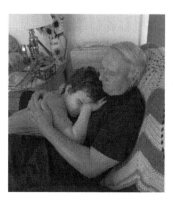

Oscar and my dad with one of Oscar's infamous snuggles.

I don't think he intentionally picks up on emotional cues but he always manages to brighten someone's day when they need it the most. It may just be a smile or giggle. If you are lucky, he will share one of his hugs with you. The best ones are the unsolicited hugs that come out of nowhere.

He gave one of those warm unsolicited hugs to a woman at my church who briefly stopped to talk to us after the Sunday service. She was sharing stories about her grandchildren who lived several states away. Oscar nonchalantly leaned into her and gave her a little side hug. She just melted. I know it was a special moment for her since she was missing her own grandchildren.

Oscar may not be able to change the world with his voice but I have no doubt that he leaves an impact on everyone he meets.

31

After spending nearly half my life working in restaurants, when it came time for me to interview for the first non-restaurant job, I was petrified. I hadn't written a resume since college and this was my first interview in decades. And while some people see time with one organization a positive, it was still alarming to view my employment history. I literally had a resume with one solitary job.

Somehow I got a call that someone was interested in setting up an interview. At this point I still had about six months of graduate school to go. It was really more of a testing-the-waters type of interview. I wasn't expecting it to go anywhere but knew I needed to practice my interview skills because it had been so long. I viewed this as a test run.

This type of job would be a life changer for my family. I could be home nights and weekends, able to take part in bath times and meals and all those things my husband had been doing on his own without complaint. Now that Oscar was in elementary school there were some days I would only see him for a few minutes.

I woke up the morning of my interview, got both boys off to where they needed to be, and enjoyed a small amount of me-time before I had to leave. My husband had left behind a note for me that I still have to this day.

He started by saying how proud he was of me and although he didn't always vocalize his support he was always my biggest cheerleader.

It was exactly what I needed and gave me a little added boost of confidence. There is something so wonderful knowing that someone loves you unconditionally. A love for your parents and your children should be a given. But when you find a partner who loves you and would do anything for you, and vice versa, it is a huge confidence booster.

That good luck note from my first interview reminds me of the strength of our family's foundation. I feel so fortunate to have found my husband and experienced that unconditional love. And yes, it would be fantastic to feel that way again. But if that is not what the future holds, so be it. I was lucky enough to experience that joy while there are others in this world who will never know what that love feels like.

HEY,

YOU ROCK THIS INTERVIEW.
YOU DESERVE IT. YOU WILL OWN IT.
REMEMBER:
YOU ARE AWESOME
YOU ARE PUT TOGETHER
    AND
YOU ARE A JONES

I WILL BE THINKING &
PRAYING FOR YOU.

THAT OUTFIT LOOKS
PROFESSIONAL AF!!
    (JUST IRON IT!)

BABE, I KNOW I SUCK AT
BACKING YOU UP, BUT I GOT
YOUR BACK. NOBODY BELIEVES
IN YOU MORE THAN ME. GO
GET THIS JOB!!
CRUSH IT!!
    ↗SORRY, HAD TO↖
I LOVE YOU ↚
WE BELIEVE IN YOU!!!

32

March 2019

The March after Wally passed away, I decided we needed a vacation. I included my parents because they had been such a huge help during the past months. I booked tickets for an indoor water park for the five of us when the boys had a three-day weekend from school. There were two bedrooms and one common area for all of us to share.

We arrived on a Saturday, checked in and spent some time at the water park. Oscar and Harvey love the water. Oscar has zero fear when it comes to going underwater which is incredibly terrifying for me. We spent that afternoon in the wave pool and slides, then went out for

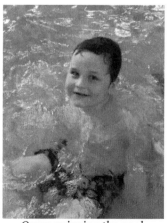

Oscar enjoying the pool, the night before his big escape.

dinner and returned to the room to relax and put the boys to bed.

The boys and I had two double beds in our room. I set Oscar up in one bed and Harvey in the other. My plan was to sleep in Harvey's bed. Since Wally had passed away, Harvey had been sleeping in my room, and I wasn't about to change things on a vacation.

I let both boys stay up a little later than usual and I went to bed at the same time as them. It had been a long day of travel and play and we were all exhausted.

Around 3:00 A.M. the phone in my room rang. It took me a few seconds to realize what the sound was. I couldn't remember the last time I had heard a phone ring in a hotel room.

Around 3:00 A.M. the phone in my hotel room rang.

The voice on the other end identified themselves as hotel security, and asked if my son was in my hotel room. Panicked, I turned on the light and realized Oscar wasn't in his bed. The phone voice told me that police officers were standing by, outside our room. The security guard described what Oscar was wearing and said he was downstairs in the arcade.

I went to the door and had to open the security deadbolt. To this day I have no idea how Oscar got out of that room. It makes no sense as we were locked inside, and the security lock was still in place, as well as the top deadbolt. I've never felt so much panic and fear for the unknown.

The police took me to the arcade where Oscar was calmly sitting in a driving game simulation, watching the cars race. When he saw me, he ran to me and I gave him the biggest hug.

The security guard explained that Oscar had been walking around the main level of the hotel. He had even walked up to a group of older kids. When they realized he couldn't talk, they told the front desk.

A security guard then followed Oscar around, thinking he might lead them back to his room. Eventually his iPad died and he handed it over to the guard hoping he could charge the battery for him. But instead, after the iPad was charged, the IT department went through all the emails on the device, eventually matching my name to the guest list.

I can't help but think someone was watching out for Oscar and our family that night. I fear for his safety often, but I never imagined something like that happening.

We have stayed in hotels since then, and I never fully get a good night's sleep. These days, by the time we are ready to go to sleep, the hotel room looks nothing like we originally found it. Furniture has been moved in front of doors to prevent my Houdini from breaking out of the room. I know this will probably be my normal for every vacation moving forward, but I will do everything I can to keep that boy safe.

33

Summer 2020

When most of the COVID-related travel bans were lifted, I decided to plan a vacation for the three of us... just Oscar, Harvey, and myself. Initially I was going to invite my parents, but at the last minute I had a moment of courage and decided the three of us would try this one on our own.

I booked flights, rental cars, and tickets for three days at Legoland in Florida, and told both boys about our trip four weeks ahead of time. Harvey was beyond excited and couldn't stop talking about vacation.

The day of our travel came but I hadn't allowed enough time to get to the airport, park, and navigate to our terminal. And I definitely didn't allow enough time to do it with two boys. We missed our flight and had to wait in the terminal for the next departure, about two hours later.

Even though it was still mid-morning, the three of us were ready to get on our way. We waited our turn to board the plane, only to be told that we could have gotten on first because of Oscar. I made a note to remember this for the return trip home.

It wasn't long into our flight before Harvey curled up in his seat and fell asleep. I was not as lucky with Oscar. He loved takeoff and landing but being confined in one spot was not for him.

A man with the food cart came by with pretzels and water. Oscar was too quick and spilled an entire tray of water onto himself and me. The flight attendant was not happy.

He reprimanded Oscar with a "Young man! That could have been hot. You can't grab trays."

I tried to apologize and explain, but he hurried off in a rage. A little while later, another flight attendant came by and saw that we were both still wet and offered extra napkins to help dry us off. I explained that Oscar was autistic and hadn't meant to spill the tray. She was so kind and told us that she used to work in a special needs classroom.

She was the first but not the last person to show us understanding on our trip. I remember her because I felt so bad that we had made a mess, and her kindness made my worries melt away.

Our three days at Legoland were fabulous. Both my boys love rides of all kinds. For most of them, Harvey needed me to sit with him due to height requirements. Oscar could sit by himself on those rides. He did so great!

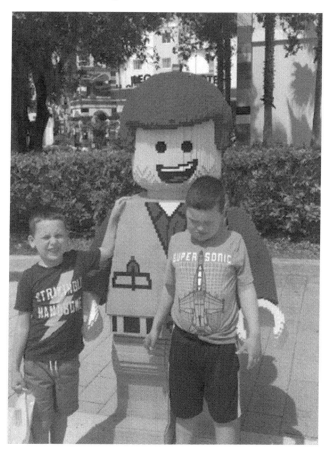

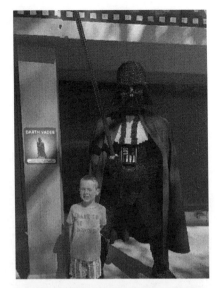

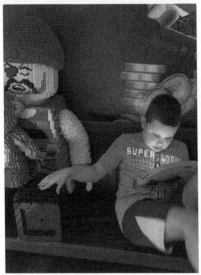

*Our trip to Legoland,
my first solo vacation with the boys.
July 2020.*

We rode all types of rides... roller coasters, water rides, and my ultimate least favorite, the round and round rides. These make me want to vomit, but every time Oscar goes on a spinning ride he laughs hysterically. I can't help but give in. They were both having so much fun that I pushed all those feelings deep down and rode all the rides.

It reminded me of when my family went to Disney World and Mom and Dad took us on every single ride that my sister and I wanted. They had never been fans of going on wild rides either.

I try to match most of my parenting skills to how my parents raised me. I think I turned out okay, and I had a very happy childhood. After all, a few spinning rides never hurt anyone.

34

Summer 2020

Trying to date in one's forties is both frustrating and disheartening. It's frustrating because I never thought I would be in this position. I missed having someone to spend time with and just be happy in their company. I also missed having someone who was excited to see me, who wanted to spend time with me, and who would make excuses to see me. It was disheartening because the older I get, the more shallow the dating pool becomes.

I mean no disrespect to the good men out there. I'm sure there are some in their forties and fifties who want to have a serious relationship, but the majority of what I have found are two types. The former has never been married. Maybe he's been engaged but at the same time he feels he's really dodged a bullet. He has no concept of a committed relationship. He's still really just out for himself. Imagine me trying to date a man like this with two boys who need a lot of attention.

The second type of guy has been married before, and for whatever reason, is now not married. Maybe his wife cheated on him. Maybe he cheated on her. Maybe they just grew out of love. Either way he is now single and has been released into the wild again. Explaining that I don't have a lot of free time after work and home life with two boys doesn't go over very well.

This second type of man only sees his kids part-time, often only on the weekends. Maybe his kids are even adults already. He doesn't want to date a woman who has younger children. If he's recently divorced, he's probably not looking for a new relationship, even if he says, "I miss being part of a couple."

Now here I come with my sad story, with my two sons and becoming a widow at the age of 42. After I told this to someone via text, they literally ceased all communication. I guess his idea of dating a widow comes with a lot of baggage. I can understand that. It does. I never stopped loving my husband. Neither of us were cheaters, and neither of us grew out of love. I'm sure that can be intimidating to someone new, especially if they think I'm comparing them to a previous great relationship.

To be fair that is exactly what I have been doing. It's exactly what I always do. When my husband and I started dating, I was blown away by how genuine he was. He called when he said he would. He apologized if he didn't text in an appropriate timeframe. Even though he lived an hour away, he still made it a point to drive to see me multiple times each week, even if it meant he didn't get as much sleep.

Within the first few weeks of dating Wally, I noticed all the differences between him and other men I had dated before. Now I notice all the qualities that are lacking from men in my current dating pool.

I would like to think that I will someday find someone to have a future with. But if that doesn't happen, I have much solace in the fact that I was fortunate to find love at least once in my life, and that it gave me my most important job—being Oscar and Harvey's mom.

35

Fall 2020

Wally and I had decided that on Harvey's first day of kindergarten we were going to take the day off and spend it together. We had planned to celebrate the fact that both our kids were in school by having a day to just be grownups. I imagine we would have done this a couple times throughout the year. A few "dates" are good for any couple.

But when that day finally arrived, I was on my own. I took the obligatory school pictures by myself. I managed to get everyone ready in plenty of time for van drivers and bus pickup. I was proud but also sad, thinking about the plans Wally and I had made so long ago.

Instead of taking a full day off from work, I opted for a half-day. I didn't feel like doing any celebrating without my husband.

My emotions got the best of me. I went to Target for a coffee and some breakfast. That was something we had liked to do as a couple. But after that I went to work.

As it turned out, Harvey didn't have the easiest time in kindergarten. He didn't want to talk about his day. He struggled with phonetics and reading but did great in math. However, he never seemed to want to do his schoolwork when he came home.

And then in March 2020, school shut down for what we were told would be "two weeks to slow the spread." The district sent home iPads with each student along with virtual learning assignments. We all hoped it was just for two weeks, but I think we parents knew this wouldn't be the case.

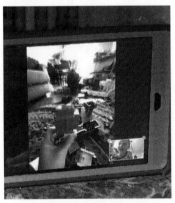

A small glimpse of what online school looks like.

We were right to second guess. Students never went back to school in the spring of 2020. Harvey was cheated out of the second half of his kindergarten year, the foundation for the next twelve years of school.

Miraculously when schools reopened in the fall of 2020, families were allowed to choose if we wanted our students to do in-person learning or virtual. I knew if Harvey did not do in-person learning, he would slip through the virtual cracks. And some sort of switch flipped for him because he loved first grade. He was excited each day. He shared about what he was doing and learning. He started doing better at reading. He continued to do great in math. Special classes were introduced, and Harvey loved art class, library, gym and music.

36

Christmas 2020

I tried my best to keep the Christmas magic alive for as long as possible for Harvey and Oscar. One of my most epic parenting fails involves the Elf on the Shelf.

The Christmas after Wally passed, to occupy Harvey, I purchased the Elf on the Shelf. Harvey named him Lego. The elf was perched on our Christmas tree until Oscar bumped into it and Lego fell out. I used two Tinker Toys to move Lego to a safe space, knowing you aren't supposed to touch him with your hands.

On Christmas Eve, the elf is supposed to go back to the North Pole. As I was putting presents under the tree and taking a bite out of a cookie left out for Santa, I tucked Lego into a kitchen drawer. My plan was to move him into a storage container later when Harvey wasn't around. But as a busy mom, that intention never came to fruition.

I had completely forgotten about Lego until the day Harvey was looking for something. It could have been bubbles or a flashlight. The possibilities are endless. But the result was the same.

"There's the elf!" Harvey screamed.

My stomach did a flip. A wave of heat took over my whole face. I tried to quickly shut the drawer but it was too late. The damage was done.

"It's because you touched him, Mom. You took away his magic and now he can't get back to the North Pole."

I felt horrible but assured Harvey that Lego was still magical. My child decided it was the fault of the closed cabinet drawer. In his seven-year-old mind, Lego was stuck because he wasn't strong enough to open the drawer from the inside.

Of course I agreed and said that must have been what happened. So three weeks after Christmas, we left the cupboard drawer open so Lego could fly home. And that is exactly what happened... according to Harvey.

Christmas magic was maintained for one more year and I learned a valuable lesson about *undecorating*.

37

Christmas 2020

Any parent who has been through Christmas vacation understands what the last few days of the year are like. You love your children and the extra time spent with them but you are very ready for them to go back to school. However, in 2020, we weren't sure if our children would ever go back to school.

Christmas and New Year's both fell on Fridays, and I was fortunate enough to not have to work. That meant two three-day weekends back to back. By the second Sunday, all of us were getting on each other's nerves.

Harvey was constantly saying, "I'm bored," and that he was already over his new toys and building sets. Oscar followed me around with a bowl or plate, just in case I didn't pick up on the fact that he wanted something to eat.

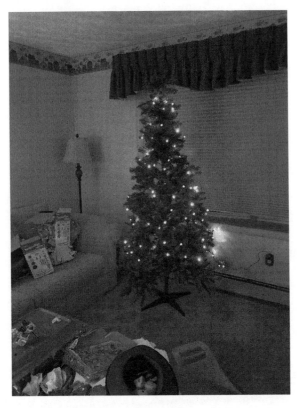

Our Christmas tree from 2020.

Oscar also stripped naked at least four times each day, just for the fun of it, while his brother Harvey made sure to notify me if I wasn't paying attention. "Oscar has his pants off. Oscar is naked now." This is frequently heard in my house on a normal day, but it seemed even more prevalent during this holiday vacation.

Sunday came to a close and I gave the boys their baths and tucked them in. I got my nightly bear hug from Oscar and played keep-away with Harvey as he tried to escape my goodnight kiss. Eventually, he popped his head out from under the covers and said, "Okay, give me a hug and a kiss and tuck me in."

After everyone was in bed and I had a minute to reflect, I decided I would take all the craziness and insane moments in order to have those snuggles, hugs, and kisses. I know our lives will never be neat and tidy, but there is a whole lot of love in our house. I remind myself that is what really matters.

38

Christmas 2020

At the end of each major holiday, either my husband or myself would announce, "Another Christmas in the books." I still say something like this to my boys when we get home from spending the day out during a holiday, almost like a pat on the back for us at the end of what was likely a stressful day.

Coming home at the end of a long holiday is always better with a partner. There is so much to unpack and unload, both physically and mentally. It's just nice to have someone to help put things away, tuck the kids in bed, clean up, and then relax together.

So here we are... Christmas 2020. My kids and I have played with Lego blocks and robots. We have made slime and tried to make crystals. Two out of the three of us have cried today. Someone lost a Lego piece and that means he will never be able to build another robot... ever, ever again.

And one of us may have cried because we felt utterly out of control. Oscar broke into the kitchen pantry one too many times. I honestly wasn't sure how to keep him occupied and safe even while doing a simple task like taking a shower.

I needed a moment. A moment to break down. Emotions got the best of me. I felt sorry for myself and my situation with no light at the end of the tunnel. Some days are harder than others, but every day has the capacity to be overwhelming. There is even more pressure on the big holidays— the Thanksgivings and Christmases and birthdays. So when those days are even a tiny bit hard, it's no wonder a parent can feel like a failure. I don't think Christmas day is ever perfect for anyone.

But if you can get to the end of the day, you are a winner. I hope what my boys remember about Christmas 2020 is how much they were loved, and not whether it was a perfect day. Looking back, I recall certain gifts, but what I really cherish is how I felt on Christmas morning and how special my parents made me feel.

That Christmas I bought Harvey a slime kit. When he opened it he said, "You didn't have to get me this. I know you hate slime." I hope this is a small little lesson for him in unconditional love.

Doing something you necessarily don't want to do isn't so bad if it makes someone you love happy. Sacrifices are easy when you have those hugs and snuggles on the other side.

39

Easter 2021

This was our third Easter without Wally. The previous year didn't really count. That was a "COVID Easter." This year we went to my mom and dad's house like we had done in the past. Oscar was comfortable there because his iPad hooked up to their Wi-Fi automatically. He also knows how to work on my dad until he is allowed to watch *Dora the Explorer* on their television.

This year my parents' house was different. They were redecorating their family room and there was no television. This didn't stop Oscar from trying to pickpocket my dad for the remote. He learned a long time ago where my dad's hiding places were. Oscar wasn't taking the lack of a television as a no.

I resorted to letting him watch his favorite videos on his iPad. We ate lunch, and I ran around after Oscar. When my nephews and Harvey went outside, Oscar wanted to follow. He got dangerously close to my mom and dad's pond and water feature.

During one party at my parents' house, Oscar had taken an opportunity to go for a swim. We both not so gracefully had fallen into the pond. So I led him back to the enclosed patio and for a little bit he was content. Then we had the Easter egg hunt and Oscar quickly learned how to snap open the plastic eggs to get to the candy.

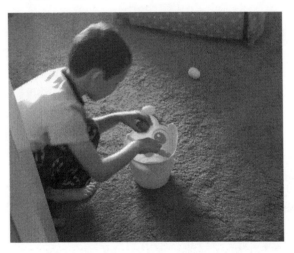

Easter morning and the hunt to find Easter baskets.

My oldest nephew announced that he wanted to get in my parents' hot tub and of course the younger boys also wanted to join in. This included Oscar. He loves any opportunity to get into water and splash around. The only problem is that he doesn't understand that he shouldn't go underwater or drink the water.

While the other boys were enjoying their soak, I tried to corral Oscar away from the hot tub. Even when everyone had exited, Oscar was still trying to get in.

The hot tub was secure and the lid was fastened tightly but Oscar's persistence led to a full meltdown. Nothing was making him happy. For a child with autism, Oscar has very few major meltdowns but when he does, they do not end until he feels like he is safe in his own space. I knew that was where this meltdown was headed.

The three of us said our goodbyes and collected our Easter baskets. Yes, *our* easter baskets. My mom lovingly still makes each of her children and their spouses and grandchildren their own Easter baskets each year.

We drove the two minutes it takes to get home. When I pulled into our driveway, I put my head on the steering wheel and took some deep breaths. It is mentally exhausting to listen to your child whimper and cry, all while trying to get them to calm down.

After a minute, Harvey asked what we were doing. I told him I just needed to take some time before we went inside. He was confused and asked again what we were doing.

I try my hardest not to lie to him and to not overly sugarcoat things, so I said, "Sometimes I just get really stressed out with your brother."

His response was, "And you miss Daddy." He knows that if he sees me cry the usual response is that I miss his father.

"Yes, I miss Daddy. Because he would have helped me today."

I miss my partner and my best friend. Everyday. But especially on the hard days. I wish he was there for the tough Harvey conversations. As Harvey gets older I can see his dad's personality. I wanted him to be there to tell me we were doing the right things for Oscar and to jump in when I wasn't feeling the most patient.

I needed those few extra minutes in the car that day to miss my husband before we all went back into the world where we were without him.

40

Spring 2021

Six months after the COVID quarantine, kids were able to return to "school" in Fall 2020. Half of the students participated in virtual learning and the rest attended regular classes. It sounded so funny to hear my first grader refer to someone in his class as a *virtual learner*.

We were almost three-quarters of the way through the school year without a COVID scare. In March our luck ran out. The first notice was for Oscar's class. His entire classroom had to be sent home and if I chose not to have him tested, he would need to stay out of school for fourteen days. The timeframe for testing began two days after exposure.

On that day we went to a close urgent care site and waited in the car for our tester. The nurse arrived in full protective gear and gave me the testing kit. In that moment I realized I would be the one doing the swabbing. This was probably the best outcome, since I'm never sure how Oscar will react to these types of things.

He handled it like a champ. He only slapped my hand away twice, which is probably less than some atypical patients.

We waited and waited. A day passed and then another. At 11:00 P.M. on the second full day I received an email that his results were ready. Even though Oscar had no symptoms, I was nervous that it would be positive. It was like taking a drug test when you know you haven't done anything wrong, but you still find yourself trying to remember if you accidently ate too many poppy seed muffins. Luckily, Oscar's results were negative and he was able to return to school the next day.

In April I received a call after work that Harvey had come in contact with a COVID-positive person. While I hadn't had to explain to Oscar what was going on, Harvey wanted to know every detail. I asked him questions about who he had been around, trying to super sleuth the identity of the person he had come into contact with who had tested positive.

He was so confused as to what his day would look like. He kept asking if I remembered how to get into all of his virtual learning sites, even though he could probably navigate to them better than me. He also questioned whether he had done something wrong. He was adamant that he hadn't touched anyone and that he had tried to keep a 6-foot distance. You have never seen anyone so diligent about following mandates. He even wore his mask until he was literally inside of our house. I assured him that he had done nothing wrong.

What a difference in the way I had to handle almost identical situations. I had a feeling that swabbing Harvey would cause more of a fight, but I was hopeful for the same negative result.

41

April 2021

I learned very early on to never discount what Oscar is capable of. I still manage to worry myself when he has something special coming up. Whether it's picture day or a doctor's appointment I always have a small level of panic for him. The outcome is almost always the same. Oscar will surprise me and will do amazing at what I consider a challenge for him.

A recent trip to the dentist was no exception. It took us until Oscar was six to find a dentist that we liked. We eventually found a pediatric dentist who also took on a lot of patients with special needs. That practice had a whole day set aside on their schedule each week just for these children.

At his first few appointments, the hygienist couldn't do the best cleaning because of how much he squirmed around. The dentist recommended a mild sedative to help him relax. I decided to give it a try and... success!

Because of the sedative, Oscar would have to miss school that day so that I could watch him and make sure there were no side effects.

Oscar still wore a little Velcro wrap around him that resembled a straight jacket, but there was no squirming. He didn't care that his hands were by his side and he couldn't be in control of his tablet. This was the first time he had an actual full and detailed cleaning.

We did this process two more times before the dentist said she thought we could try a cleaning without a sedative.

Six months later we returned for a cleaning on special needs day. Oscar was able to shimmy his hands free but the hygienist could still perform a successful cleaning. The dentist complimented me on his home care. It was so nice to hear a compliment to validate that I was doing the right things.

Flash forward to 2021. Every doctor's appointment is different since COVID. In 2021, when we arrived at the dentist we needed to call to see when we could go inside. While I did so, and went over any medical changes, I was distracted from Oscar in the back seat.

I heard him giggling and when I had a minute to look, I found Oscar with both his pants and diaper around his ankles. I ran to his side of the car and when I opened the door, Oscar quickly jumped out, thinking this was his chance to escape.

Pants at his feet, he started jumping up and down, excited to be free. There was a car parked behind us that saw the anatomy of a 9-year-old boy fairly closely. The morning commuters also had a great show. He was resistant to get back in the car and thought the whole thing was a game. His laugh was infectious and I had to laugh at the whole situation with him.

Eventually we went inside and made it to our assigned room. Oscar was put into his Velcro straight jacket. I had my phone ready so he could watch his favorite videos. There was something different about this visit. Not only did Oscar get his cleaning, he also had an electric toothbrush used and allowed the hygienist to floss. He even stayed still enough to get x-rays.

When the appointment was over, the dentist, hygienist and myself all cheered for Oscar. In return he bounced on the dentist chair with pure excitement. I hope his smile brightened their day a little and that all their patients on special needs day were as easy as Oscar.

42

March 2021

As I'm writing this, it is the eve of the 11th anniversary of my first date with Wally. It will be the third time I've had to celebrate this day without my husband.

We loved that our first date was April Fool's Day, but we never played jokes on each other. We never talked about why. It was almost an unspoken rule. We laughed with each other every day and made fun of each other often, but we never joked on April Fool's. Maybe because our marriage was already silly and fun.

As I reminisce about our first date and all the April Fool's Days that followed, I wonder how I could have ever predicted that date would turn into a wonderful family with two boys who made me laugh every day.

Oscar and Harvey are my favorite April Fools. They take after their mom and dad. I hope they always find ways to laugh throughout their life. But more than anything I hope that they find the people who make them laugh until they can't catch their breath. They have always been my favorite people. I married one of them.

43

October 2021

Three years after Wally's passing I attended my cousin's wedding, and I was prepared to shed a few tears. After all, I was someone who cried at weddings even before I lost my husband.

My mother is the only daughter in her family and has four brothers. I have nine first cousins from that side of the family. All but one of my uncles went into my grandfather's family contracting business. My mother's youngest brother became a pastor later in life. He was able to officiate during part of my husband's funeral. I had jokingly started calling him "Uncle Pastor."

I love the story of how my cousin met his wife. His father was doing work on her garage and took it upon himself to play matchmaker. My cousin was in his early 30s. A blind date was set up, the two clicked, and it was obvious that this was going to turn into a long-term relationship.

They dated for a year and announced their engagement. The wedding was planned for

Autumn of 2021. I was surprised at how excited I was to go. I wasn't sure how the boys would behave. Their last wedding was for Wally's niece and they had been much younger and easier to control then.

Uncle Pastor officiated the ceremony and it was beautiful. He touched on all the points about "finding your person" and how things happen for a reason.

I listened to the words that were meant to be joyful. It was just all too much for me. I had a ten year old sitting on my lap and an eight year old begging for the wedding to be over. And I was without my person. I was really struggling to see the reason my life had taken this turn.

My parents and Grandma sat in front of me and the boys. I don't think they noticed that I cried through the entire ceremony.

Suddenly, Oscar's patience was stretched to the limit and he no longer wanted to be sitting. Then he bit me. I tried so hard not to make any noise.

After the ceremony, Mom asked if I was okay and I answered, "No," followed by more tears. When she asked if there was anything she could do, I wasn't even thinking when I responded, "Can you cure autism?"

When cocktail hour was announced, my mom asked, "What can I get you to drink?" and she clearly did not mean a soda. My parents are not big drinkers and her asking this simple question really put things into perspective.

The reception was much less stressful than the ceremony. I was able to enjoy myself and visit with extended family. Oscar was surprisingly well behaved, and Harvey made friends with random adults, as he frequently does.

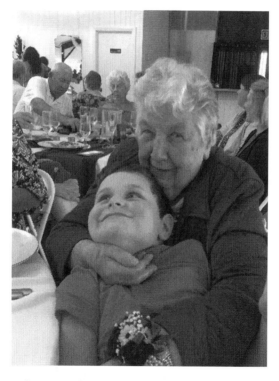

Oscar and my grandmother. They have an amazing connection.

When the bride did the traditional tossing of the bouquet, Mom asked if she could watch Oscar and if I wanted to join the single ladies to try and catch the bouquet. I quickly declined. I've come a long way in three years but I am definitely not at the standing-with-a-group-of-teenaged-girls-trying-to-catch-flowers stage yet.

44

Oscar was diagnosed with autism when he was two and a half years old. He is nonverbal and has never consistently spoken. Around the age of one he would say, "Good." And he would say it appropriately. Once in a while he would pop out another word, but it was never consistent.

He doesn't have the kind of autism where he can recite *Star Wars* lines or count cards in casinos. He's not obsessed with dinosaurs and he's not a musical prodigy.

No, Oscar's autism is a messy kind that doesn't fit perfectly into society.

There are some obvious differences at my house. There are child protectors on almost every doorknob. If Oscar gets into a room that he shouldn't be in, there's no telling what might happen. With his escape artist tendencies, I can't take a chance that he might even get out of the house.

I learned a valuable lesson about locking the refrigerator. On one occasion I left the kitchen to use the bathroom and was gone for two or three minutes. When I returned, I found every beverage placed on the kitchen island. Oscar was standing beside them with a cup in his hand.

Oscar's room has a backwards lock to keep him safe at night. My younger son knows to keep his small toys stored away because they can turn into a possible choking hazard.

Diapers are delivered to my house every month for Oscar. We have had some intermittent success with potty training, but nothing ever consistent.

Oscar looks like a typical child for his age so sometimes it's hard to explain to a stranger why he doesn't answer when asked a question. In any social situation where food is served, Oscar is on high alert. He will always seek out the person he thinks is most likely to give him food and beverages. Somehow, he recognizes the kind hearts in the world and reaches out to them in his own special way.

After nine years, I can usually predict the person in the room he will navigate toward. But my favorite Oscar interactions are the ones that take me by utter surprise with a person I never would have guessed would have the patience to endure

Oscar's persistence. It is truly amazing to see a human have this amount of warmth and understanding for my son.

45

June 2018

Every parent wants their children to experience a life equal if not better than what they had. Without being overly narcissistic, I think parents also enjoy seeing the traits that they have passed along to their kids.

Harvey has my sense of humor. I've always considered myself a funny person. I love being able to make people laugh or at least smile. I've also used humor as a defense mechanism. I realize this is not entirely a healthy way to handle adversity. I would much rather smile and laugh through the pain than to sulk and be miserable.

I remember when I realized that Harvey was going to be funnier than me. I had such an enormous sense of pride. It was like seeing your child have that achievement that was bigger and better than any success you have had in your own life.

We were running errands as a family and Wally mentioned that he could go for ice cream. I agreed with a "Me too."

And from the backseat, a four-year-old Harvey replied, "Me three."

Wally and I shared a look because we both realized that this cheesy joke and response was not something you would typically hear from a child Harvey's age.

As he's gotten older, Harvey's sense of humor has developed even more. He understands puns and uses them appropriately. He appreciates sarcasm. I can share jokes with him that I know some adults would not find funny.

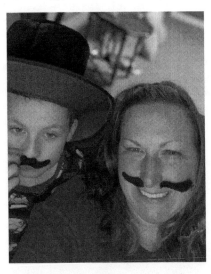

Harvey and mom bringing the moustaches back.

But most of all, like me, he is silly. He doesn't take himself too seriously and he realizes when he is able to make others laugh and enjoy themselves.

I can't take all the credit for Harvey's sense of humor. It was also one of his dad's best traits. I'm positive that Wally is enjoying all of Harvey's jokes and one liners. If Harvey is able to make me laugh this hard now, I can't wait for the jokes yet to come.

46

June 2018

Our last vacation as a family of four was to the Outer Banks in North Carolina. We had made the trip multiple times before. My parents were staying with us for the week as well. We always looked forward to our time at the beach. Then when the time came, it always went by so fast.

We had a game plan of what we wanted to accomplish other than the normal beach and pool activities. Since the boys were older this year, we decided to take a day to visit the aquarium. And while we were in that area we visited the district magistrate's office and detention center. We took a family photo to commemorate where our family originally started.

Less than five months later, my husband was gone. I had no idea that it would have been our last time at the Outer Banks. Knowing that now and looking back I would not have change anything. Both the boys had their moments with temper tantrums, but Wally and I worked well as a team to rally our troops when needed.

Eight years earlier when we had been married we invited Wally's mom and my parents. After some thought she declined. She and Wally's father had vacationed in the Outer Banks and she wanted to hold on to those memories. He had passed away five years ago.

At the time, I didn't understand but now I can definitely see her side. I am content to hold on to the memories we made there as a family even if it means I give up going to one of my favorite places.

Two years after Wally and I were married we asked his mom again to go with us on vacation as well as my parents. This time she agreed to come with us. And not even reluctantly. What changed in two years?

Oscar. That was what made the difference. She wanted to make new memories with her grandson, and see his first time at the beach. I know it was still hard for her but she was willing to put that aside to go on vacation with Oscar.

But the change in her decision really stuck with me. She knew it would be hard remembering the trip with her husband but she wanted to witness Oscar's experiences more.

I know there will be times when my own memories will be hard to bear. After years of going to the Outer Banks on family vacations, I haven't given any thought to a return trip there. I know eventually I will go back but I'm just not there.

I am at a place where I am confident that my new experiences with Oscar and Harvey will outweigh the sadness and loss that I feel everyday for their father.

Oscar & Harvey

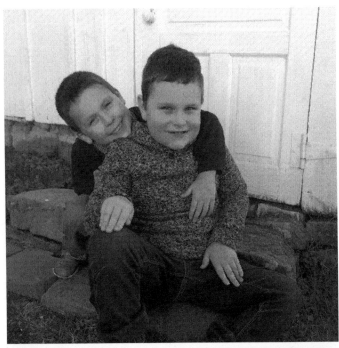

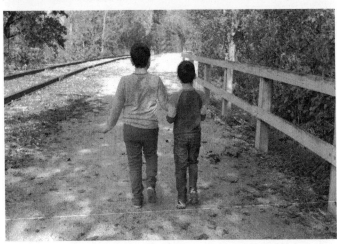

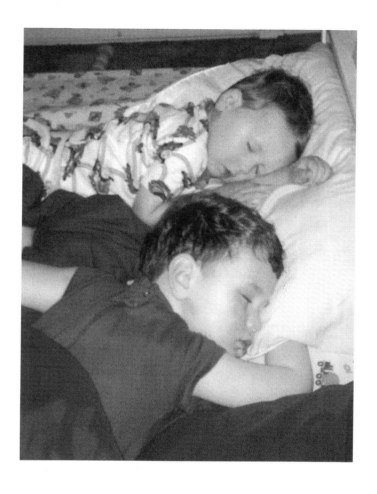

The boys with their dad.

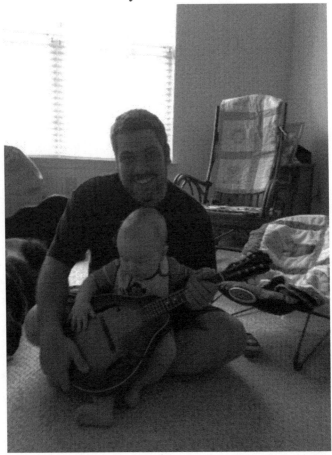

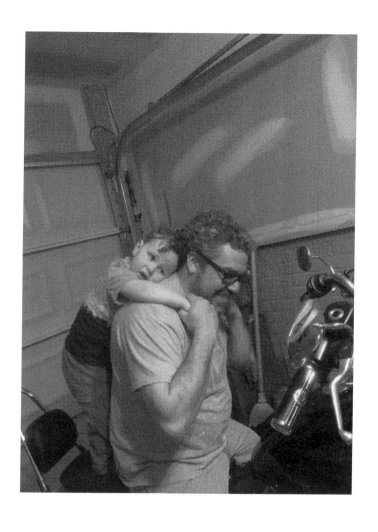

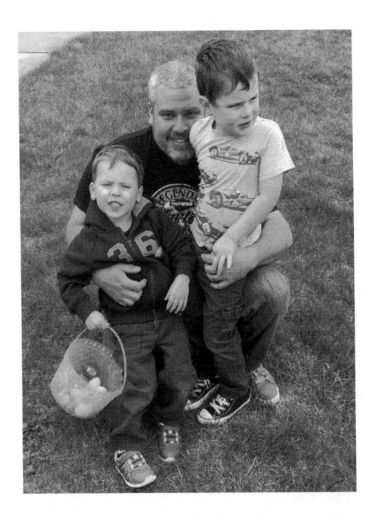

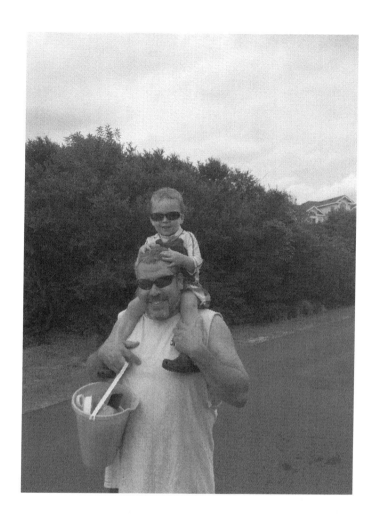

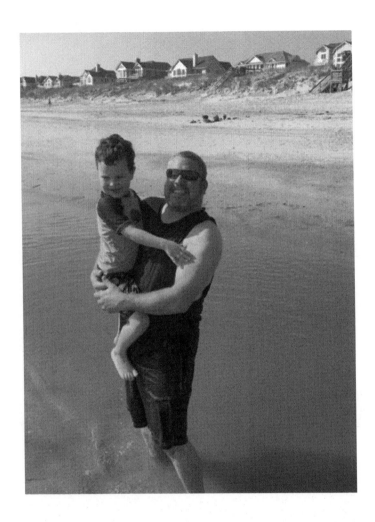

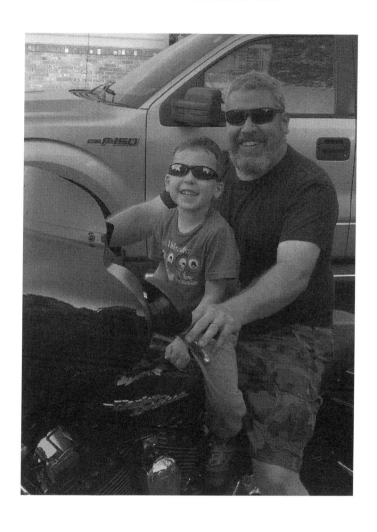

Family photos

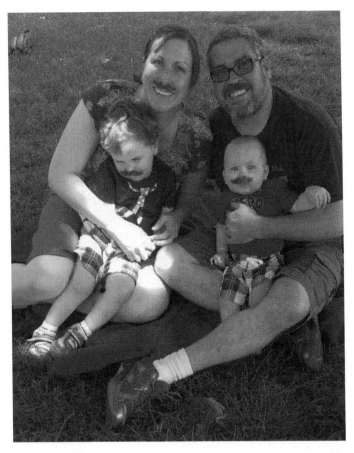

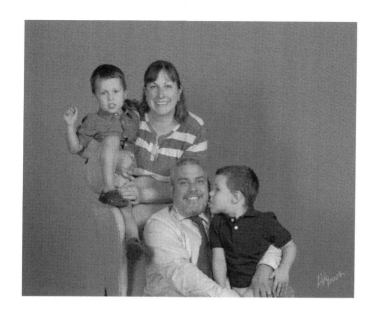

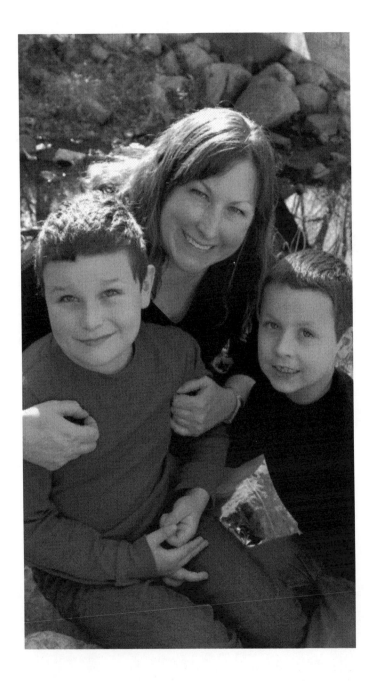

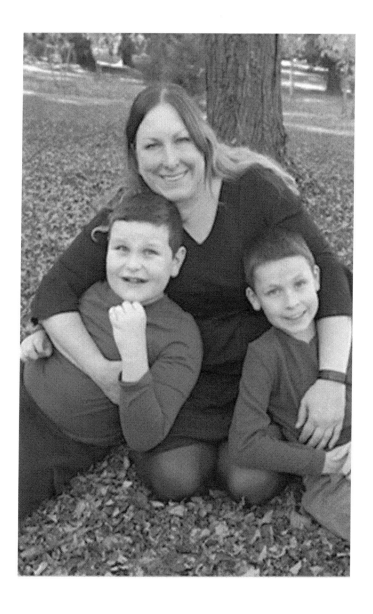

Made in the USA
Middletown, DE
25 June 2023

33323696R00118